Osteoarthritis Handbook

Osteoarthritis Handbook

Edited by

Nigel Arden MRCP MSc MD
Senior Lecturer and Consultant Rheumatologist
University of Southampton
UK

Cyrus Cooper MA DM FRCP
Professor of Rheumatology
University of Southampton
UK

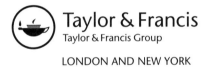

Taylor & Francis
Taylor & Francis Group

LONDON AND NEW YORK

© 2006 Taylor & Francis, an imprint of the Taylor & Francis Group

First published in the United Kingdom in 2006
by Taylor & Francis,
an imprint of the Taylor & Francis Group,
2 Park Square, Milton Park
Abingdon, Oxon OX14 4RN, UK

Tel: +44 (0) 20 7017 6000
Fax: +44 (0) 20 7017 6699
E-mail: info.medicine@tandf.co.uk
Website: http://www.tandf.co.uk/medicine

British Library Cataloguing in Publication Data

Data available on application

Library of Congress Cataloging-in-Publication Data

Data available on application

ISBN10: 1-84184-285-0

ISBN13: 9-78-1-84184-285-1

Distributed in North and South America by

Taylor & Francis
2000 NW Corporate Blvd
Boca Raton, FL 33431, USA

Within Continental USA
Tel: 800 272 7737; Fax: 800 374 3401
Outside Continental USA
Tel: 561 994 0555; Fax: 561 361 6018
E-mail: orders@crcpress.com

Distributed in the rest of the world by
Thomson Publishing Services
Cheriton House
North Way
Andover, Hampshire SP10 5BE, UK
Tel: +44 (0) 1264 332424
E-mail: salesorder.tandf@thomsonpublishingservices.co.uk

Composition by Parthenon Publishing
Printed and bound by CPI Bath, UK

Contents

Preface

Osteoarthritis is a disorder whose time has come. It is the most common joint pathology worldwide, and is a major cause of morbidity and health-care expenditure. It is timely to review the exciting new developments in this field, and to present clear guidance on evaluation and treatment for the practising clinician. Our understanding of the mechanisms that result in damage to articular cartilage and altered responsiveness of subchondral bone has grown in recent years. This has been accompanied by a better elucidation of the risk factors for osteoarthritis and the appropriate positioning of novel diagnostic technologies, such as magnetic resonance imaging (MRI) and the use of biochemical markers. Advances have also been made in the evidence base pertaining to the use of non-pharmacological and pharmacological therapeutic modalities.

The integration of these measures into a comprehensive management programme is the task of the second part of this monograph. The book will be useful to the rheumatologist, orthopaedic surgeon, general practitioner, allied health professional, and those in the pharmaceutical industry involved in the development of drugs and biological therapies for osteoarthritis. This broad constituency demands the international, multi-author contributions included herein.

Nigel Arden
Cyrus Cooper

List of contributors

Nigel Arden MRCP MSc MD
Senior Lecturer and Consultant Rheumatologist
MRC Epidemiology Resource Centre
University of Southampton
Southampton General Hospital
Tremona Road
Southampton SO16 6YD
UK

Cyrus Cooper MA DM FRCP
Professor of Rheumatology
MRC Epidemiology Resource Centre
University of Southampton
Southampton General Hospital
Tremona Road
Southampton SO16 6YD
UK

Paul Creamer MD FRCP
Consultant Rheumatologist
Directorate of Musculoskeletal Services
Southmead Hospital
Bristol BS10 5NB
UK

Anthony J Freemont MD
Professor
University of Manchester
Stopford Building
Oxford Road
Manchester M13 9PT
UK

Harry K Genant MD
Department of Radiology
Box 1250
University of California at San Francisco
San Francisco, CA 94143
USA

Kelsey M Jordan MD ChB MRCP
MRC Epidemiology Resource Centre
University of Southampton
Southampton General Hospital
Tremona Road
Southampton SO16 6YD
UK

L Stefan Lohmander MD PhD
Professor of Orthopaedic Surgery
Lund University Hospital
SE 221 85 Lund
Sweden

Andreas Mohr
Department of Diagnostic Radiology
University Hospital Schleswig-Holstein
Campus Kiel
Arnold-Heller-Strasse 9
24105 Kiel
Germany

Michael C Nevitt PhD
Professor of Epidemiology and Biostatistics
University of California at San Francisco
Prevention Sciences Group
74 New Montgomery Street
Suite 600
San Francisco, CA 94105
USA

Frank W Roemer MD
Department of Radiology
Klinikum Augsburg
Stenglinstrasse 2
86156 Augsburg
Germany

Leena Sharma MD
Associate Professor of Medicine
Department of Rheumatology
Northwestern University Medical School
303 E. Chicago Avenue
Tarry Building 3-375
Chicago, IL 60611-3008
USA

Sören Toksvig-Larsen MD PhD
Associate Professor of Orthopaedic Surgery
Lund University Hospital
SE 22185 Lund
Sweden

1

Osteoarthritis: epidemiology

Nigel Arden, Cyrus Cooper

INTRODUCTION

Osteoarthritis (OA) is the most common joint disorder in the world. In Western populations, radiographic evidence of OA can be found in the majority of people by 65 years of age, and in about 80% of those aged over 75 years. In the US, it is second only to ischaemic heart disease as a cause of work disability in men over 50 years of age, and accounts for more hospitalizations than rheumatoid arthritis (RA) each year. Despite this public health impact, OA remains an enigmatic condition to the epidemiologist. In this chapter we will review the definition and classification of OA and its prevalence, incidence and natural history.

DEFINITION AND CLASSIFICATION

Definition

The sub-division of arthritic conditions into discrete pathological entities is a relatively recent phenomenon in the history of medicine. Earlier this century, pathologists differentiated between two broad groups of arthritis: atrophic and hypertrophic. Atrophic disorders were characterized by synovial inflammation with erosion of cartilage and bone, and came to include RA and septic arthritis. The hypertrophic group was never sub-divided, however, and gradually became synonymous with what is now termed OA. The term thus encompasses a large and heterogeneous spectrum of idiopathic joint disorders.

Any working definition of OA should entail consideration of pathologic, radiologic and clinical components. The key pathological features of the disorder have been recognized for many decades, and include focal destruction of articular cartilage, followed by changes in subchondral bone. Initial post-mortem studies[1] recognized the occurrence of soft tissue changes, but emphasis was still placed on age-related degeneration of cartilage as the central feature. Subsequent pathologic and anatomic studies, mainly, but not exclusively, involving the hip joint, led to a more complex and dynamic concept of OA. The concept that OA can largely be explained as a natural reaction of synovial joints to injury and is a product of normal remodelling or repair processes in joints, stems from the work of Trueta and others,[2] and has gained considerable support from recent literature. Two other facets of the OA process have also been documented in pathological studies: synovial inflammation and crystal deposition. However, the role of these factors in disease pathogenesis remains controversial. Taken together, these studies have led to an altered concept of OA, which has developed over the last two decades and is enshrined in current approaches to definition of the disorder.[3] It is now widely viewed as an age-related dynamic reaction pattern of a joint in response to insult or injury. All tissues of the joint are involved, although the loss of articular cartilage and changes in adjacent bone remain the most striking features. In this regard, OA represents failure of the joint as an organ, analogous to renal or cardiac failure, and the pathological observations are as much a product of attempted repair as of the primary insult or damage that contributed to initiation of the process.

The radiographic features conventionally used to define OA include joint-space narrowing, osteophytes, subchondral sclerosis, cyst formation and abnormalities of bone contour. Although several radiographic grading systems have been proposed, most epidemiologic studies have utilized the Empire Rheumatism Council system, first described over three decades ago by Kellgren and Lawrence.[4] This system assigns one of five grades (0–4) to OA at various joint sites by comparison with a radiographic atlas. The criteria for increasing severity of OA are shown in Table 1.1 and relate to the assumed sequential appearance of osteophytes, joint-space loss, sclerosis and cyst. Epidemiologic studies support the notion that any radiographic grading system be joint-specific. The age- and sex-specific prevalence of OA, the individual risk factors for the disorder and the relationship between radiographic change and symptoms, are all known to differ according to joint site. There are, however, two important potential limitations of this grading system[5]: inconsistencies in the descriptions of radiographic features of OA have led to studies being performed using criteria that are discordant; furthermore, the system may place too much emphasis on the presence of osteophytes. To address these issues, recent studies have broken

Table 1.1 The Kellgren and Lawrence grading system of osteoarthritis (OA). Reproduced from Kellgren and Lawrence[4]

Radiologic features on which grades were based

Formation of osteophytes on the joint margins or, in the case of the knee joint, on the tibial spines

Periarticular ossicles; these are found chiefly in relation to the distal and proximal interphalangeal joints

Narrowing of joint cartilage associated with sclerosis of subchondral bone

Small pseudocystic areas with sclerotic walls usually situated in the subchondral bone

Altered shape of the bone ends, particularly in the head of the femur

Radiographic criteria for assessment of OA

Grade 0	None	No features of OA
Grade 1	Doubtful	Minute osteophyte, doubtful significance
Grade 2	Minimal	Definite osteophyte, unimpaired joint space
Grade 3	Moderate	Moderate diminution of joint space
Grade 4	Severe	Joint space greatly impaired with sclerosis of subchondral bone

---

up this overall radiographic grading system into its component radiographic features, quantified each feature more precisely, and assessed the reproducibility and clinical correlates of each. For the knee and hand, each of joint-space narrowing, osteophyte and the overall Kellgren and Lawrence grade show good within-observer reproducibility, with the scoring of osteophytes most closely associated with knee pain.[6,7] At the hip, however, joint-space narrowing was more reproducible than osteophyte, sclerosis or the composite score, and was the most closely associated with reported hip pain.[8] Recent atlases of standard radiographs have helped to ensure a more consistent approach to the grading of these individual features and permit greater extrapolation between the results of different studies.[9,10]

Two broad clinical areas are relevant to any definition of OA: the symptoms associated with the condition, and the degree of disability constituting its longer-term sequel. Joint pain is the dominant symptom of OA. The prevalence of joint pain rises markedly with age in the general population. However, the association between joint pain and radiographic features of OA is not constant. In studies performed during the 1950s in the north of England (Figure 1.1), the relationship between pain and radiographic evidence of OA was considerably stronger for the hip and knee than for distal interphalangeal (DIP) joint involvement.[11] Assessment of clinical outcome in OA has been the subject of intensive research in the past decade. The properties of outcome measurement

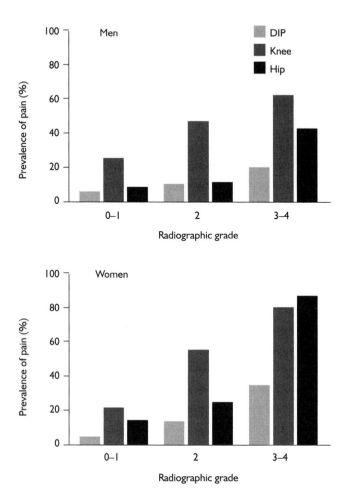

Figure 1.1 Joint symptoms and radiographic features of osteoarthritis. Data from Lawrence[11]

instruments in OA are important in determining the most appropriate methodology for studies. Reliability, validity and responsiveness to change are the three key criteria. The World Health Organization currently recommends the use of the Western Ontario and MacMaster Universities (WOMAC)[12] OA index or the Lequesne algofunctional index[13] for the monitoring of hip or knee OA. Both disease-specific instruments may be supplemented by generic health status measures, the most widely used of which are the shortform 36 (SF-36) and the Nottingham Health Profile.

Diagnostic criteria

The heterogeneity of OA has led to attempts to establish diagnostic criteria for the disorder at various joint sites. The most widely used of such criteria were developed by the American College of Rheumatology (ACR).[14,15] These criteria sets identify subjects or patients with clinical OA, using joint pain for most days of the previous month as the major inclusion parameter. This contrasts with the use of radiographic changes alone, wherein many, if not most, subjects do not report joint pain. The algorithms for classification were developed by comparing patients with clinically diagnosed OA and controls with site-specific joint pain due to other arthritic or musculoskeletal diseases. The sensitivity, specificity and accuracy of the whole range of clinical and radiographic measures in discriminating between these two groups were assessed. Table 1.2 illustrates the criteria for hand, knee and hip. The method whereby the criteria sets were derived will influence their usefulness in different settings. For clinical studies and randomized controlled trials of new interventions, selection based on the ACR criteria will enhance comparison between studies. Their use in population-based research is less clearly defined, and prevalence estimates using the ACR case definitions are likely to be substantially lower than those based on traditional radiographic criteria. Thus, the prevalence of symptomatic knee OA among women aged 45–65 years in one study was only 2.3%, in contrast with an estimate of 17% for radiographically defined disease.

Classification

Two major systems have been proposed for the classification of OA: etiologic and articular. The recognition that pathologic and radiologic features of OA could follow almost any established joint disorder led to the suggestion that OA could be classified as primary (idiopathic) or secondary. Several disorders are well recognized as causes of secondary OA. They can be divided into four main categories (Table 1.3): metabolic disorders, such as ochronosis, which lead to joint damage that can be indistinguishable from OA; anatomic derangements, such as a slipped epiphysis, which can lead to OA of the one affected joint only; major trauma or surgery to a joint, such as a meniscectomy; and a previous inflammatory arthropathy, such as RA, resulting in a secondary OA process in some of the affected joints. However, the distinction between primary and secondary OA is not always clear. For example, it has been shown that after meniscectomy, 20–25% of people will develop premature OA in the operated knee joint some 20

Table 1.2 American College of Rheumatology criteria for osteoarthritis (OA) of the hand, hip and knee

Hand	Clinical	OA is present if the items present are:
	1. Hand pain, aching or stiffness for most days of the previous month	1, 2, 3, 4 *or* 1, 2, 3, 5
	2. Hard tissue enlargement of ≥2 of 10 selected hand joints*	
	3. MCP swelling in ≤2 joints	
	4. Hard tissue enlargement of ≥2 DIP joints	
	5. Deformity of ≥1 of 10 selected hand joints	
Hip	Clinical and radiographic	
	1. Hip pain for most days of the previous month	1, 2, 3
	2. ESR ≤20 mm/h (laboratory)	*or* 1, 2, 4
	3. Radiograph femoral and/or acetabular osteophytes	*or* 1, 3, 4
	4. Radiograph hip joint-space narrowing	
Knee	Clinical	
	1. Knee pain for most days of the previous month	1, 2, 3, 4
	2. Crepitus on active joint motion	*or* 1, 2, 5
	3. Morning stiffness ≤30 min in duration	*or* 1, 4, 5
	4. Age ≥38 years	
	5. Bony enlargement of the knee on examination	
	Clinical and radiographic	
	1. Knee pain for most days of the previous month	1, 2
	2. Osteophytes at joint margins (radiograph)	*or* 1, 3, 5, 6
	3. Synovial fluid typical of OA (laboratory)	*or* 1, 4, 5, 6
	4. Age ≥40 years	
	5. Morning stiffness ≤30 min	
	6. Crepitus on active joint motion	

MCP, metacarpophalangeal joint; DIP, distal interphalangeal; ESR, erythrocyte sedimentation rate; PIP, proximal interphalangeal; CMC, carpometacarpal
* Ten selected hand joints include bilateral 2nd and 3rd PIP joints, 2nd and 3rd PIP joints and 1st CMC joints

years later,[16] although, there is also evidence that the 20% who develop secondary OA have some generalized predisposition to the disorder. Furthermore, in an individual patient it can be difficult to judge whether or not an abnormality reported many years previously is of significance to their current OA.

Table 1.3 Classification of osteoarthritis (OA)

Classification by the joints involved
Monoarticular, oligoarticular or polyarticular (generalized)
Chief joint side (index joint site) and localization within the joint
    Hip (superior pole, medial pole or concentric)
    Knee (medial, lateral, patellofemeral compartments)
    Hand (interphalangeal joints and/or thumb base)
    Spine (apophyseal joints or intervertebral disc disease)
    Others

Classification into primary and secondary forms of OA
Primary = idiopathic

Secondary indicates that a likely cause can be identified

Causes of secondary OA

    Metabolic, examples include:
        ochronosis
        acromegaly
        hemochromatosis
        calcium crystal deposition

    Anatomic, examples include:
        slipped femoral epiphysis
        epiphyseal dysplasias
        Blount's disease
        Legge–Perthe disease
        congenital dislocation of the hip
        leg length inequality
        hypermobility syndromes

    Traumatic, examples include:
        major joint trauma
        fracture through a joint or osteonecrosis
        joint surgery (e.g. meniscectomy)
        chronic injury (occupational arthropathies)

    Inflammatory, examples include:
        any inflammatory arthropathy
        septic arthritis

Classification by the presence of specific features
Inflammatory OA
    Erosive OA
    Atrophic or destructive OA
    OA with chondrocalcinosis
    Others

The second basis for sub-classifying OA relates to the number and distribution of joint sites expected. Just as there is great heterogeneity in the effects and manifestations of OA at one joint, there is variation in the pattern of joint distribution in different individuals. The condition shows a particular predilection for the DIP joint of the hand, the thumb base, the knee, the hip and the intravertebral facet joint. Involvement of more than one joint is common, and many population surveys have reported that subjects with OA in one joint have a frequency in other joints that cannot be explained by chance or age alone. Furthermore, there appear to be differences between the degree of association of OA at different joint sites. There is a stronger association between hand and knee OA, than between hip and knee disease, in Caucasian populations.[17] These differences justify the contention that OA at different sites should be treated as separate conditions.

In 1952, Kellgren and Moore described the condition of generalized OA, in which Heberden's nodes were associated with polyarticular disease.[18] The authors found that first-degree relatives of probands with generalized OA had twice the expected prevalence of multiple joint involvement, and confirmed the hereditary nature of this diathesis in a twin study. This sub-group of OA has been better characterized in recent years;[19,20] it shows a predilection for polyarticular hand involvement (particularly the interphalangeal and thumb base joints), a marked female preponderance, early inflammatory symptomatology and pronounced node formation. When large joints, for example the hip, are affected there is a tendency to diffuse (bilateral and concentric) cartilage loss. Symmetry of joint involvement in this disorder is pronounced. Generalized OA is difficult to define; it has been suggested that it means the involvement of three or more joint sites, but such definitions depend upon the age of subjects, the radiographic severity adopted for definition, the number of joint sites included in any survey, and the degree of certainty with which coincident involvement of joints on the basis of chance alone that is required.

Several other features of OA have been used in attempts to subset the disorder. For example, the term 'inflammatory OA' is sometimes used for patients with obvious inflammation and multiple joint involvement.[21] However, the joints appear to pass through phases in which this inflammation is more or less prominent, and no clear differences between patients with and without extensive inflammatory features of OA have been delineated. Some patients develop erosions of their interphalangeal joints, leading to the classification of the subset of erosive OA.[22] This disorder tends to occur in middle-aged women, presents acutely with features of inflammation and subsides over a period of months to years, leaving joint deformity and occasional ankylosis. Recent controlled data suggest that erosions in OA may simply be an aggressive form of joint destruction in a joint that is already at risk.[23] Similarly, atrophic and destructive forms of OA probably represent ends of the spectrum of disease rather than separate entities. Finally, insights into OA are provided by a variety of rare or geographically localized diseases that are associated with the development of premature disease. Examples include dysplastic conditions such as Blount's disease[24] or Mseleni disease,[25] and unusual forms of arthritis, such as Kashin–Beck disease.[25]

PREVALENCE AND INCIDENCE

Prevalence

Attempts have been made to assess the prevalence of pathologic features of OA in systematic autopsy studies. In a series of 1000 cases in 1926, Heine documented almost universal evidence of cartilage damage in people aged over 65 years. More recent studies report that cartilage erosions, subchondral reaction and osteophytes are present in the knees of 60% of men and 70% of women who die in the seventh and eighth decades of life. Prevalence estimates from such studies tend to be higher than those from radiographic surveys, partly because relatively mild pathologic change is not apparent on radiographs, and also because pathologic studies examine the whole joint surface.

Radiographic surveys of prevalence

Most currently available information on the epidemiology of OA comes from population-based radiographic surveys. In the earliest such studies, attention was focused on OA of the hand joints, or on generalized (polyarticular) OA. More recent studies from Europe and the US classify rates for individual joints and permit comparison between them.

The prevalence of radiographic OA rises steeply with age, at all joint sites. In a study from The Netherlands,[26] which included 6585 inhabitants randomly selected from the population of a Dutch village, 75% of women aged 60–70 years had OA of their DIP joints, and even by 40 years of age, 10–20% of subjects had evidence of severe radiographic disease of their hands or feet (Figure 1.2). Data from the US using the National Household Education Survey (NHES) demonstrated a prevalence of hand OA of 29.5% in subjects aged over 25 years.[27] Disease of the knee appears less frequent than that of the hand. Population-based studies in the US suggest comparable prevalence rates to those in Europe, rising from < 1% for severe radiographic disease among people aged 25–34 years, to 30% in those aged 75 years and above. Both hand and knee disease appear to be more frequent among women than men, although the female to male ratio varies among studies (between 1.5 and 4.0). Hip OA is less common than knee OA, with rates of 3–5% in the elderly population.

Prevalence of joint pain and symptomatic osteoarthritis

Although the majority of studies have focused on the prevalence of radiographic changes of OA, there is an increasing amount of research into the prevalence of knee pain in older adults in the community. This information is essential to allow accurate planning of the needs and options for the healthcare of patients. The prevalence of self-reported knee pain in the UK in adults at least 40 years of age is between 20 and 28%, with approximately 50% reporting disability as a result of their knee pain (Figure 1.3).[28] Of patients with knee pain, approximately 50% will have radiographic changes of OA, and can therefore be classified as symptomatic. Estimates from mainland Europe and the US are

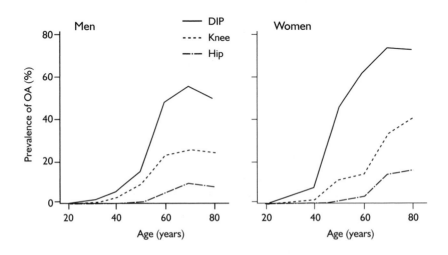

Figure 1.2 Estimates for the prevalence of radiographic osteoarthritis (OA) affecting the distal interphalangeal (DIP) joint, knee and hip in a large Dutch population sample

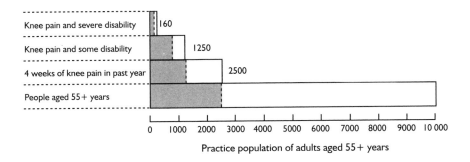

Figure 1.3 The prevalence staircase. Shading represents the proportion in each category with radiographic evidence of knee osteoarthritis. *The proportion with radiographic evidence in this category is unknown, but is likely to be high. From Cobby *et al.*[23] with permission

lower than those reported in the UK. A primary-care-based study of patients aged over 55 years from England found that 18.1% of patients registered with the practice had a clinical diagnosis of knee OA.[29] Symptomatic OA of the hip is less common than that of the knee, with prevalence estimates of between 0.7 and 4.4%, while the prevalence estimated for the hand is approximately 2.5%.

Geographic variation in prevalence

Although OA is worldwide in its distribution, geographic differences in prevalence have been reported. These are often difficult to interpret because of differences in sampling procedure and radiographic consistency. European and American data do not appear to differ markedly for hand and knee disease. However, hand involvement appears to be particularly frequent in Pima and Blackfoot Indian populations within the US. African-American females have a higher age-adjusted prevalence of knee OA than Caucasian females, but are less likely to have Heberden's nodes on physical examination.[30] Studies among African blacks in Nigeria and Liberia, as well as Jamaican blacks, confirm the lower prevalence of Heberden's nodes.[11] Greater variation has been found in the distribution of hip OA, with low rates reported among African blacks,[31] Asian Indians and Hong Kong Chinese.[32] These differences have been attributed to a lower rate of developmental hip disorders among these populations, as well as the common use of the squatting posture, which forces the hip joint through an extreme range of motion. Interestingly, despite the lower rate of hip OA, knee

OA is more common amongst Chinese women compared with Caucasian women.

Incidence

The epidemiological studies of the incidence of OA are summarized in (Table 1.4). Kallman *et al.*[33] examined hand radiographs of around 200 men in the Baltimore longitudinal study of ageing who had undergone radiography on at least four occasions over a 20-year follow-up period. They reported an incidence of radiographic OA up to 2.5–10% per year. The incidence rate rose steeply with age and was dependent on the radiographic scoring system used. The highest rates were found when using grade 1 Kellgren and Lawrence as the definition. The incidence of radiographic knee OA in the UK is estimated at 2.5% per year.[34] In a population-based incidence study of symptomatic hip and knee OA in Rochester, Minnesota, age- and sex-adjusted rates for OA of the hip and knee were found to be 47.3 per 100 000 person-years and 163.8 per 100 000 person-years, respectively.[35] The most recent data to characterize the incidence of symptomatic hand, hip and knee OA were obtained from the Fallon Community Health Plan, a health maintenance organization located in the north-east of the US[36] (Figure 1.4). In this study, the age- and sex-standardized incidence rate of hand OA was 100 per 100 000 person-years (95% CI: 86–115); for hip OA the rate was 88 per 100 000 person-years, and for knee OA the rate was 240 per 100 000 person-years. The incidence of hand, hip and knee disease increased with age, and women had higher rates than men, especially after the age of 50 years. A levelling off occurred for both groups at all joint sites around the age of 80 years. By the age of 70–89 years, the incidence of symptomatic knee OA among women

Table 1.4 Epidemiological studies of the incidence of osteoarthritis (OA)

Study	Site	Sex	Incidence rates (per 100 000)
Wilson *et al.*[35]	Hip OA	M + F	47.3
	Knee OA	M + F	163.8
Kallman *et al.*[33]	Hand OA	M	100
Oliveria *et al.*[36]	Hip OA	M + F	88
	Knee OA	M + F	240
	Hand OA	M + F	100
Cooper *et al.*[34]	Knee OA	M + F	250

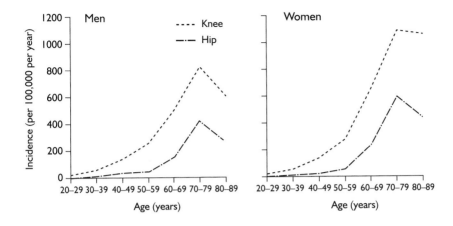

Figure 1.4 Incidence of symptomatic osteoarthritis of the hand, knee and hip. Data from the Fallon Community Health Plan[36]

approached 1% per year. Comparison of these data with age- and sex-adjusted arthroplasty rates in the northern US suggests that the rate of surgery is beginning to match the incidence rate of severe hip disease, but that a considerable short-fall exists between surgical treatment and disease incidence for knee OA.

NATURAL HISTORY

Knee osteoarthritis

Disease evolution in knee OA is slow, usually taking several years. There is emerging evidence that, once established, the condition can remain relatively stable for many years. The correlation between clinical outcome and radiographic course is relatively weak: a large study[37] demonstrated that although radiographic improvement was rare, overall clinical improvement at 1-year follow-up was common. Longer-term studies confirmed that radiographic deterioration occurs in one-third to two-thirds of patients, and that radiographic improvement is unusual (Table 1.5). A Swedish study documented that among patients with structural change, for example tibial or femoral sclerosis, the majority experienced radiographic and symptomatic deterioration over 15 years.[38] Of those subjects with only osteophytes on baseline radiography, a much smaller proportion suffered deterioration. This is broadly in accord with the

ACR Study,[39] in which joint-space narrowing was judged to be a more important determinant of progression in knee OA, than was the presence of osteophytes. However, when variables were considered in combination, this study reported that a score based on joint-space narrowing, osteophytes and sclerosis was reasonably reproducible and a better predictor of progression than any other combination.

Recent British studies[41,42] have also examined the progression of knee OA, both among subjects attending hospital outpatient departments and in the general population. In an 11-year follow-up study of 63 subjects who had baseline knee radiographs, the majority of knees did not show a worsening of the overall grade of OA, with only 33% demonstrating a deterioration in Kellgren and Lawrence score over the time period.[41] When a more sensitive global scoring system was used on paired films, the proportion showing a slight deterioration increased to 50%, and 10% showed improvement; the latter estimate is within the limits imposed by imprecision in radiographic grading. The visual analogue pain scores remained stable over the time period, but it was reported that those with knee pain at baseline had a greater chance of progressing, as did those with existing OA in the contralateral knee. A similar follow-up study was performed in 58 women aged 45–64 years from the general population, in whom unilateral knee OA (Kellgren and Lawrence grade 2 plus) had been assigned at baseline.[42]

Table 1.5 Studies of the natural history of knee osteoarthritis (OA). Modified from Dennison and Cooper[40]

Study	Subjects (n)	Measure	Follow-up (years)	Proportion deteriorated (%)
Hernborg, 1977	84 knees	C	15	55
		R	15	56
Danielsson, 1970	106 knees	R	15	33
Massardo, 1989	31	R	8	62
Dougados, 1991	353	C	1	28
		R	1	29
Schouten, 1991	142	R	12	34
Spector, 1991	63	R	11	33
Spector, 1994	58	R	2	22
Ledingham, 1995	350 knees	R	2	72
McAlindon, 1999	470	R	4	11*
Cooper et al., 2000	354	R	5	22

* Incident OA; C, clinical; R, radiographic

Follow-up radiographs at 24 months revealed that 34% of the women developed disease in the contralateral knee, and that 22% progressed radiologically in the index joint. The change in radiographic score in 354 men and women followed for 5 years is shown in Table 1.6. This demonstrates that approximately three-quarters of subjects did not progress over this time period. There remain many unanswered questions about progression of knee OA; the most important is the relationship of radiographic progression to pain, disability and the need for joint-replacement surgery.

Hip osteoarthritis

The natural history of hip OA is highly variable. Many cases that undergo surgery have a relatively short history of severe symptoms, suggesting that a progressive phase persisting between 3 months and 3 years may often precede the advanced stages of OA. There are fewer prospective studies of hip OA than of knee OA (Table 1.7). In a Danish follow-up study of 121 hips performed over three decades ago, the majority (65%) showed radiographic deterioration over a 10-year follow-up period.[43] Symptomatic improvement in this series was surprisingly common, occurring in the majority of patients. This is at variance with the results of another longitudinal study, which documented frequent deterioration in the clinical course of hip OA patients.[44] In a Dutch study of patients identified from the general population who had established OA in one or both hips, 29% showed a worsening of their radiographic scores over a 12-year follow-up

Table 1.6 Change in radiographic score of knee osteoarthritis during 5-year follow-up in 354 men and women aged 55 years or over*

Baseline K/L score	Follow-up K/L score					
	0	*1*	*2*	*3*	*4*	*All*
0	148	14	16	–	–	178
1	3	32	27	2	–	64
2	–	–	59	16	1	76
3	–	–	–	28	3	31
4	–	–	–	–	5	5
All	151	46	102	46	9	354

* The analysis was based on the worst-affected knee at baseline and follow-up[40]

Table 1.7 Studies of the natural history of hip osteoarthritis. Modified from Dennison and Cooper[40]

Study	Subjects (n)	Measure	Follow-up (years)	Proportion deteriorated (%)
Danielsson, 1964	121	C	10	19
		R	10	65
Seifert, 1969	83	C	5	83
Van Saase, 1989	86	R	12	29
Ledingham, 1993	136	C	2.3	66
		R	2.3	47

C, clinical; R, radiographic

period. Nonetheless, unlike knee OA, a few patients with hip OA experience clear-cut radiologic and symptomatic recovery;[45] this appears to occur most often among patients who have marked osteophytosis and in those with concentric disease. Osteonecrosis is the major complication of hip OA and tends to occur late in the natural history. Rapidly progressive OA can lead to an unusual appearance, with extensive bone destruction and a wide interbone distance. This appearance was initially observed among patients who ingested anti-inflammatory drugs, and was termed analgesic hip.[46,47] However, it is now recognized to occur in groups of subjects who ingest few or no such agents.

Hand osteoarthritis

OA principally affects the DIP, proximal interphalangeal (PIP) and thumb base in the hand. The evolution of hand OA is usually complete after a period of a few years. It has been studied both clinically and radiographically. The condition usually starts with aching in the affected joints, and tends to have a remitting and relapsing course over the initial years. There is often clear evidence of inflammatory phases in which individual joints become warm and tender. Bony swelling develops during this phase and cysts may form. After a variable time period, often lasting several years, these flares and the pain tend to subside. The swellings become firm and fixed, and joint movement becomes progressively reduced. The condition then appears to enter a stable phase during the seventh and eighth decades of life. Imaging studies show this evolution of change to be accompanied by sequential changes in joint anatomy and physiology. Kallman and colleagues reported that among men with DIP joint OA, more than 50% experienced progression of radiographic disease over 10 years.[33] The progression was most rapid in the DIP joints and was slower in PIP joints and the thumb base. The presence of joint-space narrowing at baseline increased the risk that subjects would develop subsequent osteophytes, and joints with severe radiographic changes at baseline had slower progression rates than joints with milder radiographic changes. The rates of OA progression in individual subjects paralleled the rate of progression hinted at by cross-sectional studies in which subjects are studied at different ages. A further 10-year follow-up study of 59 men and women with hand OA demonstrated that 48% developed new DIP osteophytes and, at either DIP, PIP or first carpometacarpal joints roughly 50% deteriorated over the period. In all, 97% of patients deteriorated when all joint scores were added together.[48]

Determinants of progression in osteoarthritis

Just as the natural history of OA differs at different joint sites, the factors that contribute to disease progression appear to be joint-specific. These determinants have been less well studied than the risk factors for prevalent disease. However, (Table 1.8) summarizes the known determinants of progression at the knee and hip.

At both sites, multiple joint involvement appears to be a determinant of accelerated disease. For example, in the French study,[16] patients who sustained joint-space narrowing in the knee over a 1-year follow-up period had a larger number of joints throughout the body affected by OA than did those who experienced no joint-space narrowing. Spector *et al.* reported that knee OA progression was more frequent in those with bilateral knee OA than in those with unilateral involvement.[21] This influence of multiple involvement extends from the knee to

Table 1.8 Determinants of progression of hip and knee osteoarthritis (OA)

	Strength of association	
Risk factor	*Knee*	*Hip*
Generalized OA diathesis	++	+
Obesity	++	+
Joint injury	++	+
Crystal deposition	+	
Neuromuscular dysfunction	+	
Knee alignment	++	
Physical activity	++	++

other joint sites. In a study of 142 subjects with baseline radiographs of the knee, Schouten and colleagues[35] found that a diagnosis of generalized OA (through the presence of Heberden's nodes) increased the likelihood of progressive cartilage loss in the knee by threefold. This increase in risk persisted after statistical adjustment for age, gender and body mass index. The co-existence of Heberden's nodes with knee OA increased the risk of knee deterioration by almost sixfold. Likewise, Doherty *et al.* found that among patients who had undergone unilateral meniscectomy previously, the presence of radiographic hand OA markedly increased the risk of developing incident knee disease.[16] The explanation for this tendency of generalized OA to increase the rate of progression is unclear; candidates include crystal deposition and a generalized hormonal or metabolic diathesis. Some studies have suggested that the presence of crystals in association with OA at baseline increases the risk of progressive disease. Thus, in one study, ten subjects with rapidly progressive OA over 1 year were compared with 84 subjects with more slowly progressive OA. The prevalence of synovial fluid crystals (hydroxyapatite or calcium pyrophosphate) was substantially higher in those with progressive disease. However, other epidemiological studies[16,35] have failed to document chondrocalcinosis as a risk factor for progression of disease, although the relatively small number of subjects with co-existent knee OA and chondrocalcinosis at baseline has limited the power of these investigations.

A further factor consistently associated with progression of OA is obesity. Several longitudinal studies[16,21,35] have reported that obese patients are more likely to experience progressive disease than non-obese patients. The evidence that weight loss slows progression of disease is less clear-cut. In the Dutch population study,[35] weight loss did not appear to slow progression. These findings contrast with the data from a clinical study of obese patients who underwent rapid weight loss, and a US epidemiological study, both of which pointed to an improvement in joint symptoms. Obesity has also been documented as a risk factor for progression in hip OA.

Other factors may influence which patients with OA experience progression. Varus or valgus alignment acts to increase medial or lateral load though the knee joint and increase the risk of disease progression four- to five-fold.[31] Other factors include muscle weakness and joint injury, which has been most convincingly demonstrated to be a determinant of progression at the knee. The relationship of growth factors or cytokines to the progression of OA needs further epidemiological and clinical investigation. Studies of insulin-like growth factor 1, a cytokine that might induce increased osteophytes over time, suggest a potential role in modifying progression. Disruption of the neurological input from structures around the joint also appears to be important in predisposing to accelerated damage. At its most extreme, this leads to the clinical phenomenon termed a Charcot joint, but lower levels of neurological disruption may lead to accelerated OA in animals.

CONCLUSIONS

OA is now firmly established as a public health problem. There have been advances in defining the disorder, measuring its component features clinically, radiographically and by using other investigative techniques. The descriptive epidemiological characteristics of OA as it affects various joint sites have been elucidated, and the risk factors for prevalent disease are clearly understood for the knee, hip and hand. Epidemiological information on the rate of progression of the disorder at these joint sites and the determinants of this progression remain less detailed. However, it is clear that progression is a joint-specific phenomenon and that there may be disease subsets at each site in which progression depends on different groups of factors. The factors that are thought to hasten progression generally include increasing age, obesity, crystal deposition, the presence of polyarticular OA, joint instability, muscle weakness and neurogenic dysfunction. The challenge of identifying subjects at risk of rapid progression through a variety of diagnostic modalities is currently the subject of intensive research. With the completion of studies examining the efficiency of biochemical markers, scintigraphy and newer imaging techniques such as magnetic resonance, it is likely that the processes underlying progressive disease will be better understood.

References

1. Collins DH. Osteoarthritis. J Bone Joint Surg Br 1953; 35-B: 518–20

2. Trueta J. Studies of the development and decay of the human frame. New York: Heinmann, 1968

3. Hutton CW. Osteoarthritis: the cause not result of joint failure? Ann Rheum Dis 1989; 48: 958–61

4. Kellgren JH, Lawrence JS. Radiological assessment of osteo-arthrosis. Ann Rheum Dis 1957; 16: 494–502

5. Spector TD, Cooper C. Radiographic assessment of osteoarthritis in population studies: whither Kellgren and Lawrence? Osteoarthritis Cartilage 1993; 1: 203–6

6. Spector TD, Hart DJ, Byrne J, et al. Definition of osteoarthritis of the knee for epidemiological studies. Ann Rheum Dis 1993; 52: 790–4

7. Kallman DA, Wigley FM, Scott WW Jr, et al. New radiographic grading scales for osteoarthritis of the hand. Reliability for determining prevalence and progression. Arthritis Rheum 1989; 32: 1584–91

8. Croft P, Cooper C, Wickham C, Coggon D. Defining osteoarthritis of the hip for epidemiologic studies. Am J Epidemiol 1990; 132: 514–22

9. Altman RD, Hochberg M, Murphy WA Jr, et al. Atlas of individual radiographic features in osteoarthritis. Osteoarthritis Cartilage 1995; 3 (Suppl A): 3–70

10. Burnett S, Hart DJ, Cooper C, Spector TD. A Radiographic Atlas of Osteoarthritis. London: Springer-Verlag, 1994: 1–45

11. Lawrence JS. Rheumatism in Populations. London: Heinemann, 1977

12. Bellamy N, Buchanan WW, Goldsmith CH, et al. Validation study of WOMAC: a health status instrument for measuring clinically important patient relevant outcomes to antirheumatic drug therapy in patients with osteoarthritis of the hip or knee. J Rheumatol 1988; 15: 1833–40

13. Lequesne MG, Mery C, Samson M, Gerard P. Indexes of severity for osteoarthritis of the hip and knee. Validation – value in comparison with other assessment tests. Scand J Rheumatol Suppl 1987; 65: 85–9

14. Altman R, Alarcon G, Appelrouth D, et al. The American College of Rheumatology criteria for the classification and reporting of osteoarthritis of the hand. Arthritis Rheum 1990; 33: 1601–10

15. Altman R, Alarcon G, Appelrouth D, et al. The American College of Rheumatology criteria for the classification and reporting of osteoarthritis of the hip. Arthritis Rheum 1991; 34: 505–14

16. Doherty M, Watt I, Dieppe P. Influence of primary generalised osteoarthritis on development of secondary osteoarthritis. Lancet 1983; 2: 8–11

17. Cushnaghan J, Dieppe P. Study of 500 patients with limb joint osteoarthritis. I. Analysis by age, sex, and distribution of symptomatic joint sites. Ann Rheum Dis 1991; 50: 8–13

18. Kellgren JH, Moore R. Generalized osteoarthritis and Heberden's nodes. Br Med J 1952; 1: 181–7

19. Egger P, Cooper C, Hart DJ, et al. Patterns of joint involvement in osteoarthritis of the hand: the Chingford Study. J Rheumatol 1995; 22: 1509–13

20. Cooper C, Egger P, Coggon D, et al. Generalized osteoarthritis in women: pattern of joint involvement and approaches to definition for epidemiological studies. J Rheumatol 1996; 23: 1938–42

21. Hart DJ, Doyle DV, Spector TD. Incidence and risk factors for radiographic knee osteoarthritis in middle aged women: the Chingford Study. Arthritis Rheum 1999; 42: 17–24

22. Utsinger PD, Resnick D, Shapiro RF, Wiesner KB. Roentgenologic, immunologic, and therapeutic study of erosive (inflammatory) osteoarthritis. Arch Intern Med 1978; 138: 693–7

23. Cobby M, Cushnaghan J, Creamer P, et al. Erosive osteoarthritis: is it a separate disease entity? Clin Radiol 1990; 42: 258–63

24. Zayer M. Osteoarthritis following Blount's disease. Int Orthop 1980; 4: 63–6

25. Sokoloff L. Endemic forms of osteoarthritis. Clin Rheum Dis 1985; 11: 187–202

26. van Saase JL, van Romunde LK, Cats A, et al. Epidemiology of osteoarthritis: Zoetermeer survey. Comparison of radiological osteoarthritis in a Dutch population with that in 10 other populations. Ann Rheum Dis 1989; 48: 271–80

27. Lawrence RC, Helmick CG, Arnett FC, et al. Estimates of the prevalence of arthritis and selected musculoskeletal disorders in the United States. Arthritis Rheum 1998; 41: 778–99

28. Peat G, McCarney R, Croft P. Knee pain and osteoarthritis in older adults: a review of community burden and current use of primary health care. Ann Rheum Dis 2001; 60: 91–7

29. Jordan KM, Sawyer S, Coakley P, et al. The use of conventional and complementary treatments for knee osteoarthritis in the community. Rheumatology (Oxford) 2004; 43: 381–4

30. Anderson JJ, Felson DT. Factors associated with osteoarthritis of the knee in the first national Health and Nutrition Examination Survey (HANES I). Evidence for an association with overweight, race, and physical demands of work. Am J Epidemiol 1988; 128: 179–89

31. Solomon L, Beighton P, Lawrence JS. Osteoarthrosis in a rural South African Negro population. Ann Rheum Dis 1976; 35: 274–8

32. Hoaglund FT, Yau AC, Wong WL. Osteoarthritis of the hip and other joints in southern Chinese in Hong Kong. J Bone Joint Surg Am 1973; 55: 545–57

33. Kallman DA, Wigley FM, Scott WW Jr, et al. The longitudinal course of hand osteoarthritis in a male population. Arthritis Rheum 1990; 33: 1323–32

34. Cooper C, Snow S, McAlindon TE, et al. Risk factors for the incidence and progression of radiographic knee osteoarthritis. Arthritis Rheum 2000; 43: 995–1000

35. Schouten JS, van den Ouweland FA, Valkenburg HA. A 12 year follow up study in the general population on prognostic factors of cartilage loss in osteoarthritis of the knee. Ann Rheum Dis 1992; 51: 932–7

36. Oliveria SA, Felson DT, Reed JI, et al. Incidence of symptomatic hand, hip, and knee osteoarthritis among patients in a health maintenance organization. Arthritis Rheum 1995; 38: 1134–41

37. Dougados M, Gueguen A, Nguyen M, et al. Longitudinal radiologic evaluation of osteoarthritis of the knee. J Rheumatol 1992; 19: 378–84

38. Hernborg J, Nillson BE. The natural course of untreated osteoarthritis of the knee. Clin Orthop 1987; 123: 130–7

39. Altman RD, Fries JF, Bloch DA, et al. Radiographic assessment of progression in osteoarthritis. Arthritis Rheum 1987; 30: 1214–25

40. Dennison E, Cooper C. The natural history and progression of osteoarthritis. In Brandt K, Doherty M, Lohmander LS, eds. Osteoarthritis, 2nd edn. Oxford: Oxford Univeristy Press, 2003: 227–33

41. Spector TD, Dacre JE, Harris PA, Huskisson EC. Radiological progression of osteoarthritis: an 11 year follow up study of the knee. Ann Rheum Dis 1992; 51: 1107–10

42. Spector TD, Hart DJ, Doyle DV. Incidence and progression of osteoarthritis in women with unilateral knee disease in the general population: the effect of obesity. Ann Rheum Dis 1994; 53: 565–8

43. Danielsson LG. Incidence and prognosis of coxarthrosis. Acta Orthop Scand 1964; 42: (Suppl): 114

44. Seifert MH, Whiteside CG, Savage O. A 5-year follow-up of fifty cases of idiopathic osteoarthritis of the hip. Ann Rheum Dis 1969; 28: 325–6

45. Bland JH, Cooper SM. Osteoarthritis: a review of the cell biology involved and evidence for reversibility. Management rationally related to known genesis and pathophysiology. Semin Arthritis Rheum 1984; 14: 106–33

46. Newman NM, Ling RS. Acetabular bone destruction related to non-steroidal anti-inflammatory drugs. Lancet 1985; 2: 11–14

47. Rashad S, Revell P, Hemingway A, et al. Effect of non-steroidal anti-inflammatory drugs on the course of osteoarthritis. Lancet 1989; 2: 519–22

48. Harris PA, Hart DJ, Dacre JE, et al. The progression of radiological hand osteoarthritis over ten years: a clinical follow-up study. Osteoarthritis Cartilage 1994; 2: 247–52

2

Risk factors for knee, hip and hand osteoarthritis

Michael C Nevitt

INTRODUCTION

Osteoarthritis (OA) is the most common form of arthritis, and one of the most frequent causes of pain, loss of function and disability in adults in Caucasian populations. The joints most frequently affected include the knees, hips and hands. Knee OA is also very common in Asian and black populations. This review of risk factors will focus primarily on the knee and hip, which are the most common sites of OA causing significant disability.

Finding risk factors for disease is important in identifying those individuals and groups who are at greatest risk, providing insights into disease etiology and suggesting ways to prevent or treat disease. The identification of high blood pressure and cholesterol as risk factors for heart disease is an informative example of how epidemiological observations on risk factors can be transformed into prevention opportunities and treatment.

DEFINITION OF OSTEOARTHRITIS

OA can be defined by structural pathology (e.g. on X-ray), joint symptoms or a combination of the two. The primary symptoms include joint pain and stiffness. Joint pathology is diverse, and includes focal damage and loss of articular cartilage, abnormal remodelling and attrition of subarticular bone, osteophytes (bone growth at the joint margins), ligamentous laxity, weakening of periarticular muscles and, in some cases, synovial distention and inflammation. Structural pathology of OA in one or more joints, as determined by radiograph or autopsy, is almost universal in the elderly.[1–3] As in many other diseases, there is only a modest correspondence in OA between pathology and symptoms.[1,4] Population studies on the frequency and determinants of OA occurrence have variously used radiographic findings of structural pathology, symptoms, a combination of radiographic findings and symptoms, or clinical diagnoses to define the disease. Even among studies evaluating structural pathology on X-ray, the criteria used to define OA often vary, including differences in the interpretation of standard grading systems, such as the Kellgren and Lawrence scales.[5] In this review, we report the results of studies without distinguishing the definition of OA used.

PREVALENCE OF KNEE, HIP AND HAND OSTEOARTHRITIS IN WESTERN EUROPE AND NORTH AMERICA

The individual joints most commonly affected by OA are the knee, hip, hand, spine and foot, with the wrists, shoulders and ankles developing OA less frequently.[4] The population impact is greatest for OA of the hips and knees, since disease is common at these sites, and pain and stiffness in large weight-bearing joints often lead to significant problems with mobility and to disability, requiring expensive surgical treatments.[6] In the US alone, the combined number of knee and hip joint replacements performed is in excess of 350 000 annually.

Using data on knee OA from a variety of population studies, Peat et al.[7] recently documented its large impact in those aged 55 years and over in Western Europe and North America. Studies have found that, on average, at any one time, radiographic findings of knee OA and frequent knee symptoms each occur in about one-quarter of people in this age group, while frequent knee symptoms and radiographic knee OA occur together in the same knee in about 12% of the population. In other words, about half of people with significant knee pain do not have radiographic OA, and about half of those with radiographic OA at any time do not have knee pain. Painful and disabling knee OA that would make an individual a candidate for total knee replacement affects at least 1 in 20 people aged 55 years and over. After the age of 70 years, radiographic knee OA has been found to occur in 40–50% of the population.[2,8] Symptomatic knee OA affects approximately 10–13% of people aged 60 years and over in the US, based on estimates from the Framingham study.[8,9] Because of its high prevalence, knee OA has a formidable impact on the older population and ranks as one of the leading causes of disability.[6]

Hip OA, whether radiographic or symptomatic, occurs less than half as frequently among adults of the same age, compared with knee OA.[10] However, owing to a lack of consensus on the best definition of radiographic hip OA,[11] estimates for X-ray disease vary from as high as 28% in people aged 45 years and over in a rural North American community[12] and 20% in the Icelandic population aged 65 years and over,[13] to as low as about 3% for the entire US population aged 55 years and older in the NHANES study.[14] It is uncertain to what extent these differences reflect true population differences versus different methods and definitions.[15]

Radiographic evidence of OA in one or more hand joints is present in about 50% of men and women by the age of 50 years, and in 75–85% by 70 years.[16–18] The distal interphalangeal (DIP) and first carpometacarpal (CMC) joints are the most commonly affected sites, followed by the proximal interphalangeal (PIP), other CMC and wrist joints. The prevalence of symptomatic hand OA is considerably lower than that of radiographic disease,[19,20] as one-third or less of radiographic hand OA is symptomatic.[17]

There are few data on the incidence of OA in populations. In the Baltimore Longitudinal Study of Aging, new OA occurred in the hand joints of men aged 60 years and over at a rate of ten affected joints per 100 person-years.[21] In a study of members of a community health plan in the Boston area, women aged 60–69 years sought care for new symptomatic hip, hand and knee OA at annual rates of 0.2, 0.4 and 0.7 per hundred, respectively.[22] Incidence rates were 25–35% lower in 60–69-year-old men.

FRAMEWORK FOR UNDERSTANDING OSTEOARTHRITIS RISK FACTORS

Epidemiological patterns in the occurrence of OA – the characteristics of those who develop the disease, which joints are affected, and at what age – provide potential clues to disease pathogenesis. A conceptual model for the pathogenesis of OA that has gained acceptance in recent years provides a framework for understanding these clues. Several important tenets of this model are: (1) cartilage, bone, muscles, ligaments and other joint tissues and structures function as a biomechanical organ system that maintains proper movement and prevents excessive joint loading; (2) systemic factors that increase overall susceptibility to joint degeneration and local biomechanical factors that impair the optimal functioning of a joint both play an important role in determining the risk of developing OA; and (3) systemic factors interact with mechanical factors operating within the local joint environment to determine which joints develop OA and how rapidly the disease progresses in an affected joint (Figure 2.1).[10,23,24]

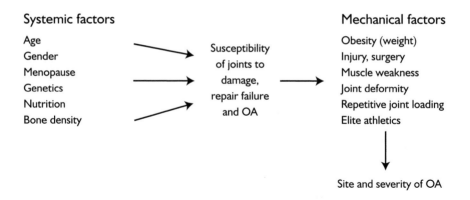

Figure 2.1 Conceptual model for the pathogenesis of osteoarthritis (OA). Adapted with permission; from Dieppe, 1995[23]

Several pathological features of OA, including proliferative bone changes, may represent attempted repair responses in an injured joint.[25] Osteophytes, for example, may result from a reactive response of cartilage and bone to abnormal mechanical loading, conferring protection to a damaged joint by reducing instability. Both systemic and local factors may operate in a joint-specific way to influence whether a reparative response is normal or aberrant, and whether it succeeds or fails in providing protection from further degeneration. The tremendous variability observed in the course of OA once it has developed[26,27] suggests a substantial role for factors influencing the biological response to damaged joint tissues. Radiographic features of OA rarely improve in appearance, but at the same time, many joints with OA remain stable radiographically over many years.[28–31] A subset of joints shows clear, often rapid, radiographic deterioration, usually accompanied by clinical evidence of worsening.[32] Even greater variability is seen in the natural course of OA symptoms, with worsening, improvement and no change occurring in similar proportions.

SYSTEMIC RISK FACTORS

A number of systemic factors have been identified as risk factors for knee, hip and hand OA. These may act by increasing the susceptibility of joints to injury, by directly damaging joint tissues, or by impairing the process of repair in damaged joint tissue.

Age and gender

All studies indicate that the prevalence and incidence of radiographic and symptomatic OA increase sharply with age.[1,8,14,16,21,22,29] This age-related increase is observed in all joints in which OA occurs, but is especially pronounced in the joints most commonly affected, such as the knee, hip and hand. As noted above, structural pathology of OA in one or more joint, as determined by radiograph or autopsy, while uncommon before the age of 40 years is nearly universal by the eighth or ninth decade. But even among the most elderly individuals, a significant proportion do not develop OA in the commonly affected joints, and some do not develop it in any joint. This suggests that OA is not an inevitable consequence of aging and that the presence of risk factors, and of specific protective factors, are important determinants of disease. Increased age is also associated with more rapid radiographic worsening of knee,[33] hip[32] and hand[34] OA in some but not all studies.

The relationship between age and the risk of OA is likely to be mediated by age-related increases in a variety of systemic and local biomechanical risk factors. Exposure to certain heavy physical activities, and occupational- and sports-related joint trauma, are notable exceptions that generally do not increase with age. Factors that do increase with age include excess joint loading from over-weight and impaired neuromuscular joint protective mechanisms (e.g. impaired muscle function and peripheral neurological responses[35–37]) and increased joint instability (e.g. ligamentous laxity[38]). Joint tissues also become more vulnerable to the effects of biomechanical insults with age. The resilience and reparative capacity of cartilage may decrease with age, owing to a reduced anabolic response to growth factors, loss of chondrocytes, and thinning of the cartilage plate.[39] It is likely that the specific local and systemic factors involved in the age-related increase in disease differ at each joint site.[24,39]

Importantly, female gender serves to amplify the age-related increase in the risk of OA occurrence in the hand, the knee and in multiple joints (so-called 'generalized OA'), so that after the age of 50 years the prevalence and incidence of disease in these joints is significantly greater in women than men.[22,40] In contrast, the frequency of hip OA increases at about the same rate with age in women and men. Hip OA appears to progress more rapidly in women[32,41] but, to date, studies have not found a gender effect on the progression of knee[29,33] or hand OA. As with age, the influence of gender on OA risk is likely to be linked to broad gender patterns in the occurrence of both systemic and local biomechanical risk factors, including hormonal differences and gender differences in obesity, body habitus, physical activity and risk of injury, muscle function[35] and joint laxity.[38] An explanation for the different gender patterns across joints will probably include an understanding of how gender-linked factors operate differently in the local environment of specific joints.[24]

Sex hormones

The accelerated age-related rise in the incidence of OA in women following menopause suggests a possible role for sex hormones, particularly oestrogen deficiency, in the systemic predisposition to OA. There is no consistent evidence linking circulating sex hormone levels[42,43] or reproductive history[44] with OA prevalence. However, many studies have examined postmenopausal oestrogen use and OA, and most,[44-49] but not all,[43,50] have found a lower prevalence or incidence of knee and hip OA in oestrogen users. Postmenopausal women using oestrogen also have larger knee cartilage volumes, assessed by magnetic resonance imaging (MRI), than non-users.[51] However, disease protection inferred from observational studies of oestrogen users may be misleading, since oestrogen use is associated with a healthy lifestyle. Oestrogen users are also more likely to have osteoporosis, which is associated with a reduced risk of OA. Evidence for a protective effect of oestrogen use is more consistent for OA defined by radiographic changes alone than for symptomatic or clinical OA,[50,52] suggesting the possibility of different effects of oestrogen on structure and symptoms. The only data from a randomized, placebo-controlled clinical trial indicated no difference in knee OA-related symptoms between women receiving oestrogen plus progestin, compared with placebo.[53]

If oestrogen deficiency has an effect on OA development or progression, a possible mechanism is its bone anti-resorptive properties in postmenopausal women, which may influence the pre-disease biomechanical environment of the joint[54] and the metabolic response of bone to excess joint loading and injury.[55] If this is the case, it is also possible that other bone anti-resorptive agents would have a similar effect. Clinical trials evaluating this possibility have recently been completed, but results to date are inconclusive.[56] Other potential mechanisms for the effect of oestrogen include direct and indirect effects on cartilage metabolism.[57]

Bone density and osteoporosis

Because reactive bone responses (subchondral bone sclerosis and osteophytes) are a prominent feature of OA pathology, there has long been an interest in the role of bone in OA initiation and progression. Cross-sectional population studies have established that women with hip or knee OA have higher bone mineral density (BMD) at skeletal sites both near to, and distant from, joints with OA.[43,58–61] Most,[43,60,62] though not all,[63] studies have found that hand OA is associated with higher BMD. High bone density is more strongly related to the presence of osteophytes than to evidence of cartilage loss.[58,61,64] These cross-sectional associations are supported by longitudinal studies that have examined skeletal status and incident knee OA.[65] In the Chingford study,[66] women with high hip or spine BMD were more likely to develop incident knee osteophytes, while women who had a fracture had a decreased risk of developing osteophytes independent of their bone density. Similarly, in the Framingham study, women with higher femoral neck bone density had an increased risk of developing new definite knee OA by the Kellgren and Lawrence scale,[67] and both women and men with high spine BMD in a longitudinal study in Baltimore were more likely to develop definite knee OA.[68] Definite knee OA by the Kellgren and Lawrence scale is defined primarily by the presence of osteophytes.

These studies describe a skeletal phenotype of high bone density that is associated with an increased risk of developing radiographic OA of the knee, hip and hand, especially when characterized by osteophytes. It has been hypothesized that subchondral trabecular microfractures from excess joint loading lead to increased subchondral bone density and stiffness, which in turn initiate the development of OA by further increasing the stresses on cartilage during joint loading.[54] Although this hypothesis suggests how higher periarticular bone density could be associated with OA, it does not provide a link between OA and overall skeletal status. Neither this hypothesis, nor the relationship between systemic and periarticular bone characteristics, have been directly evaluated in epidemiological studies, in part because non-invasive measures of periarticular bone density and biomechanical properties are technically difficult and expensive. Moreover, recent evidence from animal models indicates that cartilage lesions and degeneration precede sclerotic changes in subchondral bone.[69] Alternative explanations for the link between high bone density and the development of knee and hip OA include shared genes[64,70] and other pleiotropic factors that separately influence both bone density and OA. Obesity is strongly related to an increased risk of knee and hip OA and to high bone density, but, notably, adjustment for obesity does not account for the BMD–OA association.[43,58,60,61] Other possible common factors influencing bone density and OA include growth factors involved in both chondrogenesis and osteogenesis,[71,72] and vitamin D levels.[73]

The relationship between skeletal status and OA is complex, and the role of bone appears to differ between the initial development of OA and the course of disease once established. Detailed examination of periarticular bone in knees and hips with established OA, recently reviewed by Hunter and Spector,[55] confirm that subchondral bone is abnormal in OA, but have not revealed an elevated density or stiffness, as would be predicted by a high bone density phenotype in OA; rather, the findings indicate that subchondral bone is less stiff, more porous and has a lower mineral content and reduced biomechanical competence, compared with bone underlying joints without OA.[74] Periarticular bone in OA is metabolically active, and increased subchondral bone turnover, as indicated by bone scintigraphy, is very strongly associated with more rapid structural and clinical progression in the knee.[75] Knee subchondral bone marrow oedema-like lesions (common MRI findings in knees with OA, indicative of increased local bone turnover) are associated with abnormal joint loading and strongly predict more rapid disease progression.[76] Taken together, these studies describe important periarticular bone abnormalities in established OA, characterized by elevated turnover and remodelling, bone attrition and reduced biomechanical competence of bone underlying cartilage. Together with abnormal joint loading, these bone abnormalities may have an important role in driving structural progression.

There also appears to be a link between the behaviour of periarticular bone in progressive OA of the knee and overall skeletal status. Indeed, two longitudinal population studies suggest that structural progression of existing knee OA, including cartilage loss, is more rapid in those with low hip bone density than in those with OA who have higher bone density.[66,67] More rapid knee OA progression is also associated with faster bone loss at the hip,[67] while worsening of hand OA over time is associated with elevated metacarpal bone loss.[62] Thus, while individuals with high bone density are more likely to develop OA, progressive disease may be associated with both local and systemic osteoporosis.

Nutrition

A possible role for nutritional factors in OA is suggested by the hypothesis that OA susceptibility is increased by oxidative damage to cartilage and other joint tissues, caused by oxygen radicals that are produced by chondrocytes in damaged cartilage.[77,78] Increased intake of dietary antioxidants, such as vitamins C and E, might, therefore, protect against OA. Vitamin C is also thought to have a beneficial role in collagen synthesis.[78] One longitudinal population study found that older men and women with high dietary intakes of vitamin C had less radiographic progression of knee OA and a reduced frequency of new knee pain, but there was no association between vitamin C intake and incident radiographic findings.[78] Vitamin D status, through its important role in bone metabolism,[79] may modulate periarticular bone responses to excess loading and joint damage. Chondrocytes in OA cartilage have an increased sensitivity to vitamin D.[80] Protection against knee OA progression has been reported for older men and women with high dietary intakes, and for those with high serum levels, of vitamin D,[80] but protection from incident radiographic knee OA was not associated with vitamin D status. An increased risk of incident and progressive radiographic hip OA has been observed in elderly women with low serum levels of vitamin D.[81]

Ethnicity and race

Blacks in the US appear to have very similar overall rates of knee and hip OA, as do whites,[12,82,83] with a somewhat higher prevalence of knee OA in black than in white women, most likely attributable to a greater average body weight in the former. There is some evidence that hip OA prevalence among blacks in Africa and the Caribbean is lower than in whites.[84] A recent comparative study between Chinese and whites in the US found an equal prevalence of knee OA in men and a higher prevalence of knee OA in Chinese women, despite much lower rates of obesity in the Chinese.[85] Hand OA was about half as common and hip OA one-tenth as common in the Chinese population.[15,17] The lower risk of hip and hand OA is consistent with a lower general susceptibility for OA in the Chinese, possibly linked to genetic factors, while the contrasting and unexpectedly high prevalence of knee OA in a generally thin population may be explained by excessive knee loading from squatting[86] and other daily and occupational physical activities.

Genetics

There is good evidence indicating a genetic contribution to about half the population variability in susceptibility to hand, hip and knee OA in women,[64,87–92] and hip OA in men.[90,91] These studies suggest that multiple genes are likely to be involved in OA susceptibility and that environmental factors also have an important influence on disease expression. The evaluation of candidate genes for OA susceptibility has focused on genes encoding for type II collagen, the major form of collagen in articular cartilage, other structural proteins of the extracellular cartilage matrix, the vitamin D and oestrogen receptor genes, and bone and cartilage growth factors.[93] While results of candidate gene studies have been mixed, reasonably consistent evidence has emerged for an association of knee and multijoint OA with variations in the Col2A, VDR receptor and oestrogen receptor-α genes.[94–98] Genome-wide scans have also identified a number of promising OA susceptibility loci that point to currently unspecified genes residing on chromosomal regions that do not harbour the primary candidate genes evaluated to date.[93]

LOCAL MECHANICAL RISK FACTORS

While the systemic factors described above are hypothesized to influence susceptibility to OA in multiple joints, local biomechanical factors are thought to have a role, primarily in determining the exposure of individual joints to injury and excess loading conditions that lead to joint degeneration. Some of these biomechanical exposures are external to the joint, such as physical activities and body weight, while others, such as joint deformity, are an integral part of the local joint mechanical environment.

Obesity

Obesity is one of the strongest and best-established risk factors for knee OA,[10] clearly preceding the development of knee OA by many years,[99–101] and hastening structural worsening of existing knee OA.[30,33] There is some evidence that weight loss reduces the risk of subsequent development of knee OA.[102] As indicated by epidemiological studies of total hip replacement for OA, obesity is also a risk factor for hip OA, though less strong than for the knee.[103–105] Some,[106,107] but not all,[108] studies have also found an increased risk of hand OA in obese people. The primary mechanism for the association of obesity with knee and hip OA is likely to involve the effect of excess weight on overloading of the hip and knee joints during weight-bearing activities, causing breakdown of cartilage and damage to ligaments and other support structures.

Despite the clear role of excess joint loading in obese people as a mechanical factor in hip and knee OA, metabolic factors associated with obesity, including circulating adipocytokines, adiposity-linked glucose and lipid abnormalities and chronic inflammation, may also have a role in the pathogenesis of OA, and could explain the modest association of obesity with hand OA. Elevated levels of blood glucose[109] and C-reactive protein, a marker of inflammation that is highly correlated with obesity,[110,111] are associated with the risk of knee OA and its progression in women. It is likely that knee OA has an inflammatory component. Obesity confers a greater risk for knee OA in women than in men,[99] suggesting that in women, currently unidentified metabolic or hormonal correlates of obesity add to the effects of excess loading, to increase the risk of knee OA.

Acute injury and repetitive joint loading

Acute joint injuries, including meniscal and cruciate ligament tears in the knee, fractures and dislocations, confer a very high risk of later development of OA in the injured joint.[30,43,65,112–114] In addition to the direct effects of injury to joint tissues, disruption of normal joint mechanics and altered load distributions within the damaged joint also contribute to the long-term increased risk of subsequent OA. Severe injury may eventually cause OA in any joint, but development of disease following an acute knee injury is much more likely in individuals who have OA in another joint,[114,115] and in those with some other evidence of systemic susceptibility or who continue to stress the injured joint.[116]

Repetitive and excessive joint loading that accompanies specific physical activities and occupational tasks increases the risk of developing OA in the stressed joints. It has long been known that repetitive job tasks that require a pincer grip increase the risk of hand OA, particularly in the DIP joint.[117,118] More recently, it has been found that jobs and occupations that require kneeling, squatting, repetitive knee bending and carrying heavy loads, all activities that elevate forces across the knee and hip, substantially increase the risk of later development of knee[119–121] and hip OA.[122,123] Excess body weight is likely to amplify the effects of knee-bending activities on the risk of knee OA.[120]

Moderate recreational running and sports participation do not appear to increase the risk of hip or knee OA, independently of joint injuries that may be suffered in the course of these activities.[116] However, elite and professional athletes engaged in sports involving high-impact forces directly to joints and torsional joint loading are at substantially increased risk of subsequent development of OA in the affected joints, even without major injury. An increased risk of knee or hip OA has been found in former elite soccer players, runners and American-football players.[116,124–127]

Joint deformity

Congenital abnormalities that result in abnormal load distributions within the joint, such as acetabular dysplasia and slipped capital femoral epiphysis of the hip, are associated with a very high risk of later development of OA in the affected joint.[128] Whether common subclinical joint malformations, such as mild acetabular dysplasia, increase the risk of hip OA is uncertain.[128] One prospective study found that reduced acetabular coverage in older women increased the risk of subsequently developing hip OA,[129] but several cross-sectional studies have not found an association between hip OA and measures of subclinical acetabular dysplasia, in either men or women.[130,131]

The mechanical alignment of the knee, as indicated by the hip/knee/ankle angle, is an important determinant of load distribution in the knee during ambulation, with a more varus alignment associated with greater loads in the medial compartment and a more valgus alignment with greater loads in the lateral compartment.[132] Varus and valgus malalignment are found with much greater frequency in knees with evidence of OA involvement in the medial and lateral compartments, respectively.[76] Malalignment in knees with advanced OA results, in part, from progressive loss of cartilage and subchondral bone in the involved compartment and degeneration of supporting structures (e.g. ligamentous laxity), and appears to contribute to a vicious cycle of further damage to cartilage and bone in the compartment subjected to increased loads.[24] OA knees with a varus malalignment have a 3–4-fold increased risk of further joint-space narrowing in the medial compartment, while OA knees with a valgus malalignment have a similarly increased risk of further lateral compartment joint-space narrowing.[133] Subchondral bone marrow oedema-like lesions are much more likely to occur in a knee compartment that is subjected to increased loads due to a mechanical malalignment (i.e. medial compartment lesions in varus knees).[76] These subchondral lesions probably represent injury to bone due to the abnormal loading and to focal damage to the overlying cartilage, and may be an important driver of further cartilage loss in the involved compartment.

It is biomechanically plausible that mild knee-alignment deformities precede and contribute to the initial development of knee OA, but this has not yet been evaluated in longitudinal studies. Even in a normally aligned knee, 60–70% of the weight-bearing load is transmitted through the medial compartment,[132] which may explain a strong predilection for medial compartment involvement in knees with OA.[134]

Muscle strength and weakness

Greater muscle contraction forces increase joint loads during activity. Consistent with this, increased grip strength in men is associated with a greater risk of developing OA in the PIP, metacarpophalangeal and first CMC joints, which are the hand joints subjected to the greatest forces during grip.[135] On the other hand, co-contraction of quadriceps and hamstrings during gait functions to attenuate loads in the knee, suggests that greater strength in these muscles might confer some protection against the development of knee OA. Consistent with this, one longitudinal study found that quadriceps weakness increased the risk of subsequent development of radiographic knee OA in women;[136] however, other prospective data to support this protective effect are lacking.

Knees with existing OA have weaker quadriceps than knees without OA, especially when symptoms are present (probably due to disuse atrophy), but weakness is also present in knees without pain or evidence of muscle atrophy (possibly due to arthrogenous inhibition of muscle contraction).[137] Whether greater quadriceps strength can protect against further progression of knee OA is uncertain. One study found that stronger quadriceps were not associated with reduced progression of knee OA.[138] In contrast, a recent, more-detailed examination of this question found that stronger quadriceps were associated with a greater progression of existing OA in knees that had a compromised biomechanical environment, specifically in knees with a varus or valgus malalignment and knees with medial lateral laxity.[139] Thus, whether increased muscle strength can protect against further progression of knee OA may depend on other local factors that influence load distribution.

CONCLUSIONS

Existing data from epidemiological studies on risk factors for knee, hip and hand OA are consistent with a model for OA pathogenesis in which systemic factors influence the underlying susceptibility of multiple different joints to tissue damage and repair failure, while local mechanical factors, both external and intrinsic to the joint, determine the site of joint degeneration and severity of the disease (Figure 2.1). Although many potential risk factors have not been systematically evaluated for associations with OA at multiple joint sites, consistent associations with knee, hip and hand OA have been observed for several systemic risk factors, such as age, bone density and family history (Table 2.1). However,

Table 2.1 Risk factors for knee, hip and hand osteoarthritis (OA)

Risk or protective factor	Knee OA Prevalent and/or incident	Knee OA Progressive	Hip OA Prevalent and/or incident	Hip OA Progressive	Hand AO Prevalent and/or incident	Hand AO Progressive
Increased age	+ +	+	+ +	+	+ +	+
Female gender	+ +			+ +	+ +	?
Sex hormone levels		?	?	?		?
Postmenopausal HRT	– –	–	–	?	–	?
High BMD	+ +	–	+ +	?	+ +	–
High vitamin C intake		–	?	?	?	?
High vitamin D intake/levels		–	–	–	?	?
Black African descent	+	?	–	?	?	?
Chinese descent	+	?	– –	?	–	?
Family history/ inheritance	+ +	?	+ +	?	+ +	?
Obesity	+ +	+ +	+ +		+	?
Acute joint injury	+ +		+ +	?	+ +	?
Occupational repetitive joint loading	+ +	?	+ +	?	+ +	?
Elite athletes in contact sports	+ +	?	+ +	?	?	?
Joint deformity	?	+ +	+ +	?	?	?
Muscle strength	–	+	?	?	+	?

+ +, Strong evidence of increased risk; +, moderate evidence of increased risk; no entry, evidence suggests no effect; –, moderate evidence of protective effect; – –, strong evidence of protective effect; ?, insufficient or conflicting evidence; HRT, hormone replacement therapy; BMD, bone mineral density

there are informative exceptions, such as female gender, which is associated with a greater risk of knee and hand OA but not hip OA.

Many risk factors probably act through both local mechanical and systemic pathways. Age, for example, has effects on the risk of OA through multiple pathways, which include systemic declines in cartilage anabolic and repair capacity, as well as local mechanical pathways, such as declining periarticular muscle function and increasing joint laxity.[24,39] It is also likely that there are joint-specific characteristics of cartilage metabolism that modulate the susceptibility of different joints to systemic influences, to a greater or lesser extent. For example, findings from one recent study suggest that chondrocytes in knee and ankle cartilage respond differently to environmental stimuli, in terms of suppression of matrix synthesis and increased catabolic activity.[140] Genetic factors are also very likely to have both joint-specific mechanical effects, for example by encoding for anatomic variations that influence the biomechanics of each joint, and also systemic effects on the function and metabolism of cartilage and other joint tissues.[141]

Local mechanical factors, almost by definition, have a high degree of joint specificity, such as acetabular dysplasia for hip OA and mechanical knee alignment for knee OA. (Obesity may be an interesting exception in that, although acting primarily through local mechanical pathways (joint loading), it may also have systemic effects through metabolic/hormonal correlates of obesity.) It is likely that additional local mechanical factors will be identified that extend our understanding of the site-specific nature of OA risk – this is likely to include identification of different determinants of disease in each of the three compartments of the knee, reflecting the unique biomechanics of each compartment,[142] as well as for different joints of the hand. Prolonged squatting, for example, is associated with an increased risk of medial and lateral tibiofemoral OA, but not patellofemoral OA, in Chinese women.[86]

Some evidence has emerged that is suggestive of the interplay between specific systemic and local factors, which will be important for accurately estimating the risk of developing OA. A potential example of this is the finding in several studies of an increased risk of developing knee OA following a meniscal injury when the injury occurs in an individual who has, or develops, hand OA (a likely marker of genetic susceptibility to OA), compared with a meniscal injury in a person without hand OA. Another possible example is the apparently greater effect of obesity on the risk of knee OA in women in comparison to men, which may reflect the combined effects of excess joint loading and systemic susceptibility related to postmenopausal hormonal status and metabolic correlates of obesity itself. Large prospective cohort studies are needed further to investigate and describe such interactions, which may be useful in identifying individuals who will benefit most from specific preventive interventions and treatments.[143]

The existing studies also suggest that there may be distinct risk-factor profiles for the onset of OA and for its progression, which, if true, would provide insights about disease biology and have implications for prevention. The most notable example of this from the present review is the observation that bone density has opposite effects on knee OA progression compared with incidence, with high bone density protecting against joint-space narrowing in knees with OA, but also increasing the risk of developing early disease characterized by osteophytes.[66,67] As another example, greater quadriceps strength may protect against the initial development of knee OA,[136] but either has no effect[138] or may even increase the risk of disease progression.[139] Other studies suggest that vitamin D and vitamin C deficiencies increase the risk of progressive but not incident radiographic knee OA.[78] Finally, a recent cohort study examining multiple risk factors found that obesity, hand OA, previous knee injury and regular participation in outdoor sports increased the risk of newly occurring knee OA, but only obesity significantly affected the risk of progressive disease.[30] Some differences in the effect of risk factors on incident versus progressive OA may reflect different roles in bone proliferation, a radiographic marker of early OA, versus progressive cartilage loss. Even so, preventive strategies may need to be tailored to the risk factors implicated in each stage of disease development.

In summary, a variety of risk factors have been found that are useful in identifying those with the greatest risk of developing OA, especially knee OA, and, among those with OA, individuals with a high risk of progressive disease. Some of the strongest and best-established risk factors, including older age, female gender, congenital joint malformation, prior knee injury (once it has occurred) and a family history of OA, are not themselves amenable to modification. However, these characteristics may still be useful for targeting those most in need of prevention and treatment. Being overweight or obese is a strong risk factor for knee and hip OA, and amenable to intervention. However, weight loss programmes, in general, are usually only modestly successful and recidivism is high. Fortunately, recent investigations have begun to identify some potentially modifiable risk factors, including bone density and, possibly, periarticular bone turnover, varus and valgus malalignment of the knee, certain types of physical activities and sports injuries, and dietary factors, all of which may lead to effective avenues for future treatments and prevention.

References

1. Lawrence JS, Bremner JM, Bier F. Osteo-arthritis: prevalence in the population and relationship between symptoms and X-ray changes. Ann Rheum Dis 1966; 25: 1–23

2. Bagge E, Bjelle A, Edén S, Svanborg A. Osteoarthritis in the elderly: clinical and radiological findings in 79 and 85 year olds. Ann Rheum Dis 1991; 50: 535–9

3. Cole AA, Margulis A, Kuettner KE. Distinguishing ankle and knee articular cartilage. Foot Ankle Clin 2003; 8: 305–16, x

4. Dieppe P. Osteoarthritis. Acta Orthop Scand 1998; 281 (Suppl): 2–5

5. Spector TD, Cooper C. Radiographic assessment of osteoarthritis in population studies: Whither Kellgren and Lawrence? Osteoarthritis Cartilage 1993; 1: 1–4

6. Guccione AA, Felson DT, Anderson JJ, et al. The effects of specific medical conditions on the functional limitations of elders in the Framingham Study. Am J Public Health 1994; 84: 351–8

7. Peat G, McCarney R, Croft P. Knee pain and osteoarthritis in older adults: a review of community burden and current use of primary health care. Ann Rheum Dis 2001; 60: 91–7

8. Felson DT, Naimark A, Anderson J, et al. The prevalence of knee osteoarthritis in the elderly. Arthritis Rheum 1987; 30: 914–18

9. Felson DT, Zhang Y. An update on the epidemiology of knee and hip osteoarthritis with a view to prevention. Arthritis Rheum 1998; 41: 1343–55

10. Felson DT, Lawrence RC, Dieppe PA, et al. Osteoarthritis: new insights. Part 1: the disease and its risk factors. Ann Intern Med 2000; 133: 635–46

11. Nevitt MC. Definition of hip osteoarthritis for epidemiological studies. Ann Rheum Dis 1996; 55: 652–5

12. Jordan JM, Linder GF, Renner JB, Fryer JG. The impact of arthritis in rural populations. Arthritis Care Res 1995; 8: 242–50

13. Ingvarsson T, Haagglund G, Lohmander LS. Prevalence of hip osteoarthritis in Iceland. Ann Rheum Dis 1999; 58: 201–7

14. Lawrence RC, Helmick CG, Arnett FC, et al. Estimates of the prevalence of arthritis and selected musculoskeletal disorders in the United States. Arthritis Rheum 1998; 41: 778–99

15. Nevitt MC, Xu L, Zhang Y, et al. Very low prevalence of hip osteoarthritis among Chinese elderly in Beijing, China, compared with whites in the United States: the Beijing osteoarthritis study. Arthritis Rheum 2002; 46: 1773–9

16. Van Saase JLCM, Van Romunde LKJ, Cats A, et al. Epidemiology of osteoarthritis: Zoetermeer survey. Comparison of radiological osteoarthritis in a Dutch population with that in 10 other populations. Ann Rheum Dis 1989; 48: 271–80

17. Zhang Y, Xu L, Nevitt MC, et al. Chinese in Beijing have a lower prevalence of hand osteoarthritis than whites in Framingham, MA. Arthritis Rheum 2004; in press

18. Bagge E, Bjelle A, Valkenburg HA, Svanborg A. Prevalence of radiographic osteoarthritis in two elderly European populations. Rheumatol Int 1992; 12: 33–8

19. Cushnaghan J, Dieppe P. Study of 500 patients with limb joint osteoarthritis. I. Analysis by age, sex and distribution of symptomatic joint sites. Ann Rheum Dis 1991; 50: 8–31

20. Zhang Y, Niu J, Kelly-Hayes M, et al. Prevalence of symptomatic hand osteoarthritis and its impact on functional status among the elderly: The Framingham Study. Am J Epidemiol 2002; 156: 1021–7

21. Kallman D, Wigley F, Scott W. The longitudinal course of hand osteoarthritis in a male population. Arthritis Rheum 1990; 33: 1323–32

22. Oliveria SA, Felson DT, Reed JI, et al. Incidence of symptomatic hand, hip, and knee osteoarthritis among patients in a health maintenance organization. Arthritis Rheum 1995; 38: 1134–41

23. Dieppe P. The classification and diagnosis of osteoarthritis. In Kuettner KE, Goldberg VM, eds. Osteoarthritic Disorders. Rosemont, IL: American Academy of Orthopedic Surgeons, 1995: 5–12

24. Sharma L. Local factors in osteoarthritis. Curr Opin Rheumatol 2001; 13: 441–6

25. Dieppe P. Subchondral bone should be the main target for the treatment of pain and disease progression in osteoarthritis. Osteoarthritis Cartilage 1999; 7: 325–6

26. Felson DT. The course of osteoarthritis and factors that affect it. Rheum Dis Clin North Am 1993; 19: 607

27. Dieppe P, Cushnagen J. The natural course and prognosis of osteoarthritis. In Moskowitz RW, ed. Osteoarthritis: Diagnosis and Medical/Surgical Management. Philadelphia: WB Saunders, 1992: 399–412

28. Hernborg JS, Nilsson BE. The natural course of untreated osteoarthritis of the knee. Clin Orthop 1977; 123: 130–7

29. Felson DT, Zhang Y, Hannan MT, et al. The incidence and natural history of knee osteoarthritis in the elderly. The Framingham Osteoarthritis Study. Arthritis Rheum 1995; 38: 1500–5

30. Cooper C, Snow S, McAlindon TE, et al. Risk factors for the incidence and progression of radiographic knee osteoarthritis. Arthritis Rheum 2000; 43: 995–1000

31. Lachance L, Sowers MF, Jamadar D, Hochberg M. The natural history of emergent osteoarthritis of the knee in women. Osteoarthritis Cartilage 2002; 10: 849–54

32. Dougados M, Gueguen A, Nguyen M, et al. Radiological progression of hip osteoarthritis: definition, risk factors and correlations with clinical status. Ann Rheum Dis 1996; 55: 356–62

33. Schouten JSAG, van den Ouweland FA, Valkenburg HA. A 12 year follow up study in the general population on prognostic factors of cartilage loss in osteoarthritis of the knee. Ann Rheum Dis 1992; 51: 932–7

34. Busby J, Tobin J, Ettinger W, et al. A longitudinal study of osteoarthritis of the hand: the effect of age. Ann Hum Biol 1991; 18: 417–24

35. Newman AB, Haggerty CL, Goodpaster B, et al. Strength and muscle quality in a well-functioning cohort of older adults: the Health, Aging and Body Composition Study. J Am Geriatr Soc 2003; 51: 323–30

36. Hurley MV. The role of muscle weakness in the pathogenesis of osteoarthritis. Rheum Dis Clin North Am 1999; 25: 283–98, vi

37. Sharma L. Proprioceptive impairment in knee osteoarthritis. Rheum Dis Clin North Am 1999; 25: 299–314, vi

38. Sharma L, Lou C, Felson DT, et al. Laxity in healthy and osteoarthritic knees. Arthritis Rheum 1999; 42: 861–70

39. Loeser RF, Shakoor N. Aging or osteoarthritis: which is the problem? Rheum Dis Clin North Am 2003; 29: 653–73

40. Kellgren JH, Moore R. Generalized osteoarthritis and Heberden's nodes. Br Med J 1952; 1: 181–7

41. Ledingham J, Dawson S, Preston B, et al. Radiographic progression of hospital referred osteoarthritis of the hip. Ann Rheum Dis 1993; 52: 263–7

42. Cauley J, Kwoh C, Egeland G, et al. Serum sex hormones and severity of osteoarthritis of the hand. J Rheumatol 1993; 20: 1170–5

43. Sowers MF, Hochberg M, Crabbe JP, et al. Association of bone mineral density and sex hormone levels with osteoarthritis of the hand and knee in premenopausal women. Am J Epidemiol 1996; 143: 38–47

44. Samanta A, Jones A, Regan M, et al. Is osteoarthritis in women affected by hormonal changes or smoking? Br J Rheumatol 1993; 32: 366–70

45. Hannan MT, Felson DT, Anderson JJ, et al. Oestrogen use and radiographic osteoarthritis of the knee in women. Arthritis Rheum 1990; 33: 525–32

46. Nevitt MC, Cummings SR, Lane NE, et al. Current use of oral oestrogen is associated with a decreased prevalence of radiographic hip OA in elderly white women. Arthritis Rheum 1994; 37 (Suppl): S212

47. Spector TD, Nandra D, Hart DJ, Doyle DV. Is hormone replacement therapy protective for hand and knee osteoarthritis in women? The Chingford Study. Ann Rheum Dis 1997; 56: 432–4

48. Zhang Y, McAlindon TE, Hannan MT, et al. Oestrogen replacement therapy and worsening of radiographic knee osteoarthritis: the Framingham Study. Arthritis Rheum 1998; 41: 1867–73

49. Hart D, Doyle D, Spector T. Incidence and risk factors for radiographic knee osteoarthritis in middle-aged women: the Chingford Study. Arthritis Rheum 1999; 42: 17–24

50. Oliveria SA, Felson DT, Klein RA, et al. Oestrogen replacement therapy and the development of osteoarthritis. Epidemiology 1996; 7: 415–19

51. Wluka AE, Davis SR, Bailey M, et al. Users of ooestrogen replacement therapy have more knee cartilage than non-users. Ann Rheum Dis 2001; 60: 332–6

52. Nevitt MC, Felson DT. Sex hormones and the risk of osteoarthritis in women: epidemiological evidence. Ann Rheum Dis 1996; 55: 673–6

53. Nevitt MC, Felson DT, Williams EN, Grady D. The effect of oestrogen plus progestin on knee symptoms and related disability in postmenopausal women: The Heart and Oestrogen/Progestin Replacement Study, a randomized, double-blind, placebo-controlled trial. Arthritis Rheum 2001; 44: 811–18

54. Radin EL, Paul IL, Rose RM. Role of mechanical factors in pathogenesis of primary osteoarthritis. Lancet 1972; 1: 519–22

55. Hunter DJ, Spector TD. The role of bone metabolism in osteoarthritis. Curr Rheumatol Rep 2003; 5: 15–19

56. Spector TD. Bisphosphonates: potential therapeutic agents for disease modification in osteoarthritis. Aging Clin Exp Res 2003; 15: 413–18

57. Sowers MF. Oestrogens and osteoarthritis: hormone replacement, menopause and aging. In Lobo RA, Kelsey J, Marcus R, eds. Menopause: Biology and Pathobiology. New York: Academic Press, 2000: 274–90

58. Hannan MT, Anderson JJ, Zhang Y, et al. Bone mineral density and knee osteoarthritis in elderly men and women: The Framingham Study. Arthritis Rheum 1993; 36: 1671–80

59. Dequeker J, Boonen S, Aerssens J, Westhovens R. Inverse relationship osteoarthritis-osteoporosis: what is the evidence? What are the consequences? Br J Rheumatol 1996; 35: 813–18

60. Hart D, Mootooswamy I, Doyle D, Spector T. The relationship between osteoarthritis and osteoporosis in the general population: the Chingford Study. Ann Rheum Dis 2004; in press

61. Nevitt MC, Lane NE, Scott JC, et al. Radiographic osteoarthritis of the hip and bone mineral density. Arthritis Rheum 1995; 38: 907–16

62. Sowers M, Zobel D, Weissfeld L, et al. Progression of osteoarthritis of the hand and metacarpal bone loss. Arthritis Rheum 1991; 34: 36–42

63. Hochberg MC, Lethbridge-Cejku M, Scott WW, et al. Appendicular bone mass and osteoarthritis of the hands in women: data from the Baltimore Longitudinal Study of Aging. J Rheumatol 1994; 21: 1532–6

64. MacGregor AJ, Antoniades L, Matson M, et al. The genetic contribution to radiographic hip osteoarthritis in women: results of a classic twin study. Arthritis Rheum 2000; 43: 2410–16

65. Sowers M, Lachance L, Jamadar D, et al. The associations of bone mineral density and bone turnover markers with osteoarthritis of the hand and knee in pre- and perimenopausal women. Arthritis Rheum 1999; 42: 483–9

66. Hart DJ, Cronin C, Daniels M, et al. The relationship of bone density and fracture to incident and progressive radiographic osteoarthritis of the knee: the Chingford Study. Arthritis Rheum 2002; 46: 92–9

67. Zhang Y, Hannan MT, Chaisson CE, et al. Bone mineral density and risk of incident and progressive radiographic knee osteoarthritis in women: the Framingham Study. J Rheumatol 2000; 27: 1032–7

68. Hochberg MC, Lethbridge-Cejku M, Tobin JD. Bone mineral density and osteoarthritis: data from the Baltimore Longitudinal Study of Aging. Osteoarthritis Cartilage 2004; 12 (Suppl A): S45–8

69. Dedrick DK, Goldstein SA, Brandt KD, et al. A longitudinal study of subchondral plate and trabecular bone in cruciate-deficient dogs with osteoarthritis followed up for 54 months. Arthritis Rheum 1993; 36: 1460–7

70. Antoniades L, MacGregor AJ, Matson M, Spector TD. A cotwin control study of the relationship between hip osteoarthritis and bone mineral density. Arthritis Rheum 2000; 43: 1450–5

71. Dequeker J, Mohan S, Finkelman RD, et al. Generalized osteoarthritis associated with increased insulin-like growth factor types I and II and transforming growth factor β in cortical bone from the iliac crest. Arthritis Rheum 1993; 36: 1702–8

72. Hammerman D, Stanley RE. Implications of increased bone density in osteoarthritis. J Bone Miner Res 1996; 11: 1205–8

73. Lane NE, Gore LR, Cummings SR, et al. Serum vitamin D levels and incident changes of radiographic hip osteoarthritis: a longitudinal study. Study of Osteoporotic Fractures Research Group. Arthritis Rheum 1999; 42: 854–60

74. Ding M, Odgaard A, Hvid I. Changes in the three-dimensional microstructure of human tibial cancellous bone in early osteoarthritis. J Bone Joint Surg Br 2003; 85: 906–12

75. Dieppe P, Cushnaghan J, Young P, Kirwan J. Prediction of the progression of joint space narrowing in osteoarthritis of the knee by bone scintigraphy. Ann Rheum Dis 1993; 52: 557–63

76. Felson DT, McLaughlin S, Goggins J, et al. Bone marrow oedema and its relation to progression of knee osteoarthritis. Ann Intern Med 2003; 139: 330–6

77. Sowers M, Lachance L. Vitamins and arthritis. The roles of vitamins A, C, D, and E. Rheum Dis Clin North Am 1999; 25: 315–32

78. McAlindon TE, Jacques P, Zhang Y, et al. Do antioxidant micronutrients protect against the development and progression of knee osteoarthritis? Arthritis Rheum 1996; 39: 648–56

79. Parfitt AM, Gallagher JC, Heaney RP, et al. Vitamin D and bone health in the elderly. Am J Clin Nutr 1982; 36: 1014–31

80. McAlindon TE, Felson DT, Zhang Y, et al. Relation of dietary intake and serum levels of vitamin D to progression of osteoarthritis of the knee among participants in the Framingham Study. Ann Intern Med 1996; 125: 353–9

81. Lane NE, Gore, LR, Cummings SR, et al. Serum vitamin D levels and incident changes of radiographic hip osteoarthritis: a longitudinal study. Study of Osteoporotic Fractures Research Group. Arthritis Rheum 1999; 5: 854–60

82. Anderson JJ, Felson DT. Factors associated with osteoarthritis of the knee in the first national health and nutrition examination survey (Hanes I). Am J Epidemiol 1988; 128: 179–89

83. Tepper S, Hochberg MC. Factors associated with hip osteoarthritis: data from the First National Health and Nutrition Examination Survey (NHANES–I). Am J Epidemiol 1993; 137: 1081–8

84. Lawrence JS, Sebo M. The geography of osteoarthritis. In Kent NG, ed. The Aetiopathogenesis of Osteoarthritis. Baltimore: University Park Press, 1980: 155–83

85. Zhang Y, Xu L, Nevitt MC, et al. Comparison of the prevalence of knee osteoarthritis between the elderly Chinese population in Beijing and whites in the

United States: The Beijing Osteoarthritis Study. Arthritis Rheum 2001; 44: 2065–71

86. Zhang Y, Hunter DJ, Nevitt MC, et al. Association of squatting with increased prevalence of radiographic tibiofemoral knee osteoarthritis: the Beijing Osteoarthritis Study. Arthritis Rheum 2004; 50: 1187–92

87. Spector TD, Cicuttini F, Baker J, et al. Genetic influences on osteoarthritis in women: a twin study. Br Med J 1996; 312: 940–3

88. Kaprio J, Kujala UM, Peltonen L, Koskenvuo M. Genetic liability to osteoarthritis may be greater in women than men. Br Med J 1996; 313: 232

89. Felson DT, Couropmitree NN, Chaisson CE, et al. Evidence for a Mendelian gene in a segregation analysis of generalized radiographic osteoarthritis: the Framingham Study. Arthritis Rheum 1998; 41: 1064–71

90. Lanyon P, Muir K, Doherty S, Doherty M. Assessment of a genetic contribution to osteoarthritis of the hip: sibling study. Br Med J 2000; 321: 1179–83

91. Ingvarsson T, Steffansson SE, Hallgrimsdottir IB, et al. The inheritance of hip osteoarthritis in Iceland. Arthritis Rheum 2000; 43: 2785–92

92. Jonsson H, Manolescu I, Stefansson SE, et al. The inheritance of hand osteoarthritis in Iceland. Arthritis Rheum 2003; 48: 391–5

93. Loughlin J. Genetic epidemiology of primary osteoarthritis. Curr Opin Rheumatol 2001; 13: 111–16

94. Keen RW, Hart DJ, Lanchbury JS, Spector TD. Association of early osteoarthritis of the knee with a Taq I polymorphism of the vitamin D receptor gene. Arthritis Rheum 1997; 40: 1444–9

95. Meulenbelt I, Bijkerk C, De Wildt SC, et al. Haplotype analysis of three polymorphisms of the COL2A1 gene and associations with generalised radiological osteoarthritis. Ann Hum Genet 1999; 63: 393–400

96. Uitterlinden AG, Burger H, van Duijn CM, et al. Adjacent genes, for COL2A1 and the vitamin D receptor, are associated with separate features of radiographic osteoarthritis of the knee. Arthritis Rheum 2000; 43: 1456–64

97. Ushiyama T, Ueyama H, Inoue K, et al. Oestrogen receptor gene polymorphism and generalized osteoarthritis. J Rheumatol 1998; 25: 134–7

98. Bergink AP, van Meurs JB, Loughlin J, et al. Oestrogen receptor alpha gene haplotype is associated with radiographic osteoarthritis of the knee in elderly men and women. Arthritis Rheum 2003; 48: 1913–22

99. Felson DT, Zhang Y, Hannan M, et al. Risk factors for incident radiographic knee osteoarthritis in the elderly. Arthritis Rheum 1997; 40: 728–33

100. Spector TD, Hart DJ, Doyle DV. Incidence and progression of osteoarthritis in women with unilateral knee disease in the general population: the effect of obesity. Ann Rheum Dis 1994; 53: 565–8

101. Gelber AC, Hochberg MC, Mead LA, et al. Body mass index in young men and the risk of subsequent knee and hip osteoarthritis. Am J Med 1999; 107: 542–8

102. Felson DT, Zhang Y, Anthony JM, et al. Weight loss reduces the risk of symptomatic knee osteoarthritis in women. Ann Intern Med 1992; 116: 535–9

103. Karlson EW, Mandl LA, Aweh GN, et al. Total hip replacement due to osteoarthritis: the importance of age, obesity, and other modifiable risk factors. Am J Med 2003; 114: 93–8

104. Vingard E, Alfredsson L, Malchau H. Lifestyle factors and hip arthrosis. A case referent study of body mass index, smoking and hormone therapy in 503 Swedish women. Acta Orthop Scand 1997; 68: 216–20

105. Cooper C, Inskip H, Croft P, et al. Individual risk factors for hip osteoarthritis: obesity, hip injury, and physical activity. Am J Epidemiol 1998; 147: 516–22

106. Carman WJ, Sowers M, Hawthorne VM, Weissfeld LA. Obesity as a risk factor for osteoarthritis of the hand and wrist: a prospective study. Am J Epidemiol 1994; 139: 119–29

107. Oliveria SA, Felson DT, Cirillo PA, et al. Body weight, body mass index, and incident symptomatic osteoarthritis of the hand, hip, and knee. Epidemiology 1999; 10: 161–6

108. Hochberg MC, Lethbridge-Cejku M, Scott WW Jr, et al. Obesity and osteoarthritis of the hands in women. Osteoarthritis Cartilage 1993; 1: 129–35

109. Hart DJ, Doyle DV, Spector TD. Association between metabolic factors and knee osteoarthritis in women: the Chingford Study. J Rheum 1995; 22: 1118–23

110. Spector TD, Hart DJ, Nandra D, et al. Low-level increases in serum C-reactive protein are present in early osteoarthritis of the knee and predict progressive disease. Arthritis Rheum 1997; 40: 723–7

111. Sowers M, Jannausch M, Stein E, et al. C-reactive protein as a biomarker of emergent osteoarthritis. Osteoarthritis Cartilage 2002; 10: 595–601

112. Gelber AC, Hochberg MC, Mead LA, et al. Joint injury in young adults and risk for subsequent knee and hip osteoarthritis. Ann Intern Med 2000; 133: 321–8

113. Roos H, Lauren M, Adalberth T, et al. Knee osteoarthritis after meniscectomy: prevalence of radiographic changes after twenty-one years, compared with matched controls. Arthritis Rheum 1998; 41: 687–93

114. Englund M, Paradowski PT, Lohmander LS. Association of radiographic hand osteoarthritis with radiographic knee osteoarthritis after meniscectomy. Arthritis Rheum 2004; 50: 469–75

115. Doherty M, Watt I, Dieppe P. Influence of primary generalized osteoarthritis on development of secondary osteoarthritis. Lancet 1983; 7: 8–11

116. Buckwalter JA, Lane NE. Athletics and osteoarthritis. Am J Sports Med 1997; 25: 873–81

117. Lawrence J. Rheumatism in cotton operatives. Br J Ind Med 1961; 18: 270–6

118. Hadler NM, Gillings DB, Imbus HR, et al. Hand structure and function in an industrial setting: influence of three patterns of stereotyped, repetitive usage. Arthritis Rheum 1978; 21: 210–20

119. Felson DT, Hannan MT, Naimark A, et al. Occupational physical demands, knee bending and knee osteoarthritis: results from the Framingham Study. J Rheumatol 1991; 18: 1587–92

120. Coggon D, Croft P, Kellingray S, et al. Occupational physical activities and osteoarthritis of the knee. Arthritis Rheum 2000; 43: 1443–9

121. Cooper C, McAlindon T, Coggon D, et al. Occupational activity and osteoarthritis of the knee. Ann Rheum Dis 1994; 53: 90–3

122. Croft P, Cooper C, Wichham C, Coggon D. Osteoarthritis of the hip and occupational activity. Scand J Work Environ Health 1992; 18: 59–63

123. Thelin A. Hip joint arthrosis: an occupational disorder among farmers. Am J Ind Med 1990; 18: 339–43

124. Vingard E, Alfredsson L, Goldie I, Hogstedt C. Sports and osteoarthrosis of the hip. An epidemiologic study. Am J Sports Med 1993; 21: 195–200

125. Kujala UM, Kaprio J, Sarna S. Osteoarthritis of weight bearing joints of lower limbs in former elite male athletes. Br Med J 1994; 308: 231–4

126. Kujala UM, Kettunen J, Paananen H, et al. Knee osteoarthritis in former runners, soccer players, weight lifters and shooters. Arthritis Rheum 1995; 38: 539–46

127. Spector TD, Harris PA, Hart DJ, et al. Risk of osteoarthritis associated with long-term weight-bearing sports: a radiologic survey of the hips and knees in female ex-athletes and population controls. Arthritis Rheum 1996; 39: 988–95

128. Harris WH. Etiology of osteoarthritis of the hip. Clin Orthop Rel Res 1986; 213: 20–33

129. Lane NE, Lin P, Christiansen L, et al. Association of mild acetabular dysplasia with an increased risk of incident hip osteoarthritis in elderly white women: the study of osteoporotic fractures. Arthritis Rheum 2000; 43: 400–4

130. Smith RW, Egger P, Coggon D, et al. Osteoarthritis of the hip joint and acetabular dysplasia. Ann Rheum Dis 1995; 54: 179–81

131. Lane NE, Nevitt MC, Cooper C, et al. Acetabular dysplasia and osteoarthritis of the hip in elderly white women. Ann Rheum Dis 1997; 56: 627–30

132. Andriacchi TP. Dynamics of knee malalignment. Orthop Clin North Am 1994; 25: 395–403

133. Sharma L, Song J, Felson DT, et al. The role of knee alignment in disease progression and functional decline in knee osteoarthritis. J Am Med Assoc 2001; 286: 188–95

134. Felson DT, Nevitt MC, Zhang Y, et al. High prevalence of lateral knee osteoarthritis in Beijing Chinese compared with Framingham Caucasian subjects. Arthritis Rheum 2002; 46: 1217–22

135. Chaisson CE, Zhang Y, Sharma L, et al. Grip strength and the risk of developing radiographic hand osteoarthritis: results from the Framingham Study. Arthritis Rheum 1999; 42: 33–8

136. Slemenda C, Heilman DK, Brandt KD, et al. Reduced quadriceps strength relative to body weight: a risk factor for knee osteoarthritis in women? Arthritis Rheum 1998; 41: 1951–9

137. Slemenda C, Brandt KD, Heilman DK, et al. Quadriceps weakness and osteoarthritis of the knee. Ann Intern Med 1997; 127: 97–104

138. Brandt KD, Heilman DK, Slemenda C, et al. Quadriceps strength in women with radiographically progressive osteoarthritis of the knee and those with stable radiographic changes. J Rheumatol 1999; 26: 2431–7

139. Sharma L, Dunlop DD, Cahue S, et al. Quadriceps strength and osteoarthritis progression in malaligned and lax knees. Ann Intern Med 2003; 138: 613–19

140. Cole AA, Kuettner KE. Molecular basis for differences between human joints. Cell Mol Life Sci 2002; 59: 19–26

141. Spector TD, MacGregor AJ. Risk factors for osteoarthritis: genetics. Osteoarthritis Cartilage 2004; 12 (Suppl A): S39–44

142. Cicuttini FM, Spector T, Baker J. Risk factors for osteoarthritis in the tibiofemoral and patellofemoral joints of the knee. J Rheumatol 1997; 24: 1164–7

143. Felson DT, Nevitt MC. Epidemiologic studies for osteoarthritis: new versus conventional study design approaches. Rheum Dis Clin North Am 2004; 30: 783–97

3

Diagnosis of osteoarthritis

Frank W Roemer, Andreas Mohr, Harry K Genant

INTRODUCTION

The term osteoarthritis (OA) summarizes a group of degenerative joint disorders characterized by loss of articular cartilage, alterations of subchondral bone and osteophyte formation. Together with clinical symptoms and findings, radiography has been the main technique used to diagnose OA and assess disease progression. However, as radiography provides only a record of rather advanced changes of OA, it is insensitive to initial alterations and minor disease progression. Advances in disease-modifying treatments for OA have led to an increased demand for superior imaging methods, particularly magnetic resonance imaging (MRI), to measure therapeutic efficacy.

The focus of this chapter is to provide an overview of the different imaging modalities, with an emphasis on newer imaging methods such as MRI and computed tomography (CT). Clinical and laboratory findings are also covered.

CLINICAL FEATURES

The diagnosis of OA is largely based on obtaining a detailed history and conducting a complete physical examination. Ancillary diagnostic tests may be necessary when the diagnosis remains uncertain.

Pain is usually the first and cardinal symptom of OA involving only one or a few joints. Typically, pain progresses gradually over time, increases with weight bearing and is usually relieved by rest in the early course of the disease. Symptoms progress to constant pain on use of the affected joint and, finally, with more advanced joint involvement, pain occurs at rest and at night. Pain may be localized to the joint or it may be referred, such as lumbar facet joint degeneration resulting in pain in the buttock or OA of the hip presenting as pain in the knee. Cold, damp weather tends to exacerbate the symptoms, although pain is sometimes aggravated by heat.

Morning stiffness is common and characteristically resolves within 1 hour, depending on severity. Stiffness may also occur following periods of inactivity. As the disease progresses, prolonged joint stiffness is evident, and is probably due to a combination of joint incongruity and capsular fibrosis. In contrast to rheumatoid arthritis, stiffness in OA is confined to the affected joint. Loss of function is specific to the site involved, for example restricted walking distance, limp and fatigue in OA of the hip and knee, or poor grip in cases of OA of the hand.

Musculoskeletal examination may reveal signs of inflammation,[1] swelling, deformities, joint enlargement, crepitus[2] and limitation of motion. Muscle spasm, and tendon and capsular contracture may also be observed, depending on the site and duration of involvement.

The American College of Rheumatology have developed clinical, or combined clinical and radiographic, classification criteria for the diagnosis of OA of the knee, hand and hip.[3–5] Table 3.1 shows a summary of the classification

Table 3.1 Criteria for classification of idiopathic osteoarthritis (OA) of the knee[3]

Clinical and laboratory	Clinical and radiographic	Clinical
Knee pain	Knee pain	Knee pain
+ at least 5 of 9:	+ at least 1 of 3:	+ at least 3 of 6:
Age > 50 years	Age > 50 years	Age > 50 years
Stiffness < 30 minutes	Stiffness < 30 min	Stiffness < 30 min
Crepitus	Crepitus	Crepitus
Bony tenderness	+ Osteophytes	Bony tenderness
Bony enlargement		Bony enlargement
No palpable warmth		No palpable warmth
ESR < 40 mm/hour		
RF < 1:40		
SF OA		
92% sensitive	91% sensitive	95% sensitive
75% specific	86% specific	69% specific

ESR, erythrocyte sedimentation rate (Westergren); RF, rheumatoid factor; SF OA, synovial fluid signs of OA (clear, viscous, or white blood cell count < 2000/mm^3)

criteria for knee OA using clinical and laboratory data, clinical and radiographic information, or clinical examination only. A sensitivity of 91% and specificity of 86% can be achieved with a combination of clinical and radiological criteria.[3] For classification of symptomatic OA of the hands, three out of four clinical criteria, such as pain, hard tissue enlargement or deformity, have to be present to classify a patient as having OA of the hand (Table 3.2).[4]

A classification rule for symptomatic hip OA was developed by applying a combination of clinical and radiographic criteria. The best rule required hip pain with at least two of three of the following criteria: erythrocyte sedimentation rate < 20 mm/h, radiographic evidence of osteophytes and/or evidence of joint-space narrowing (Table 3.3).[5]

None of the criteria for classification of disease are perfect, but it is hoped that they will help facilitate the uniform reporting of OA of the knee, hands and hip in future studies.

Table 3.2 Clinical classification criteria for osteoarthritis of the hand[4]

Hand pain, aching or stiffness and 3 or 4 of the following features:
Hard-tissue enlargement of 2 or more of 10 selected joints
Hard-tissue enlargement of 2 or more DIP joints
Fewer than 3 swollen MCP joints
Deformity of at least 1 of 10 selected joints*

*The 10 selected joints are the second and third distal interphalangeal (DIP), the second and third proximal interphalangeal, and the first carpometacarpal joints of both hands. This classification method yields a sensitivity of 94% and a specificity of 87%.
MCP, metacarpophalangeal

Table 3.3 Combined clinical (history, physical examination, laboratory) and radiographic classification criteria for osteoarthritis of the hip[5]

Hip pain and at least 2 of the following 3 features:
ESR < 20 mm/h
Radiographic femoral or acetabular osteophytes
Radiographic joint-space narrowing (superior, axial and/or medial)

This classification method yields a sensitivity of 89% and a specificity of 91%.
ESR, erythrocyte sedimentation rate (Westergren)

IMAGING

Radiography

Radiographic findings provide objective evidence of disease. These findings may include the presence of joint-space narrowing, osteophyte formation, pseudo-cysts and sclerosis of subchondral bone. Complications of the disease, such as loose bony bodies and ankylosis, are also depicted well. Many patients with radiographic changes consistent with OA are asymptomatic or do not exhibit any disability, suggesting that the presence of radiographic changes in the absence of symptoms should not lead to the diagnosis of OA. On the other hand, the absence of radiographic changes does not exclude the diagnosis of OA.

There are drawbacks to the use of plain radiography for the diagnosis and evaluation of OA: radiologic evaluation is relatively insensitive in depicting early changes, and a follow-up period of at least 1 year is needed to assess disease progression; conventional radiographs provide detailed images of cortical and trabecular bone, but cannot directly visualize the articular cartilage or other non-calcified structures of the affected joint; and, although osseous findings are common in OA, they tend to arise late in the disease process, and may be secondary consequences of chondral, meniscal or ligamentous changes. Furthermore, radiography projects a three-dimensional anatomy onto a two-dimensional image, which results in morphological distortion, magnification and superimposition of overlying structures. However, radiography remains a readily available and cost-efficient tool for the diagnosis of OA, and usually serves as a sufficient basis for clinical and therapeutic decisions.

Technical considerations

Since OA is a progressive disease, it is important to use radiographic procedures that are easily reproducible. Assessment of joint-space width can only be made when opposing articular surfaces are in direct contact, which may necessitate weight bearing of the joint to displace any intervening fluid.[6]

In the knee, mild flexion optimizes contact between the affected regions of the joint. As intra-articular cartilage loss is non-homogeneous, small changes in the position of a joint may be a source of bias when measuring the joint-space width on serial examinations.[7] Suggestions for improving the reproducibility of positioning in radiography of the knee joint have been made. The semi-flexed metatarsophalangeal (MTP) technique[8,9] and the fixed-flexion technique[10] seem to be superior to fluoroscopic semi-flexed radiography[11,12] for reproducibility in

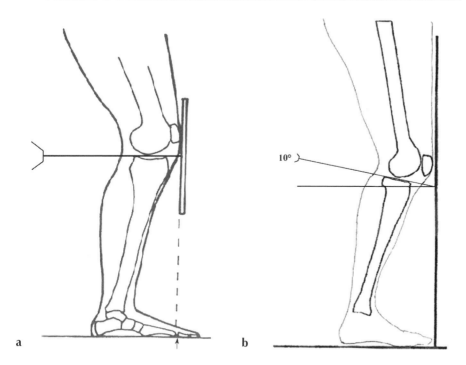

Figure 3.1 Radiography of knee osteoarthritis. Semi-flexed metatarsophalangeal (MTP) and fixed-flexion technique. (a) Semi-flexed or MTP position (posterior–anterior (PA) view). 15° external rotation of the foot. The first MTP joint of the foot is aligned below and in line with the front edge of the film cassette (arrow). 7–10° flexion of the knee. The anterior surface of the knee touches the cassette. Image adapted from reference 8. (b) Fixed-flexion radiography of the knee (PA view). 10° external rotation of the foot while the toes are touching the vertical table. Knees and thighs touching the table for support. The X-ray beam is angled 10° caudal and centred on the joint line. Adapted from reference 10

joint-space measurements in longitudinal trials (Figure 3.1). In order to assess the load line and alignment of the knee joint – important prognostic parameters for disease progression and functional decline – whole-leg films are necessary.[13]

Joint-space narrowing

In contrast to the inflammatory arthritic disorders, cartilage loss in OA is usually circumscribed, and tends to involve the part of the joint exposed to the greatest mechanical stress, such as the superolateral aspect of the hip or the medial femoro-tibial space of the knee. Exceptions to this focal cartilaginous destruction are found in OA of the interphalangeal joints of the hands (Figure

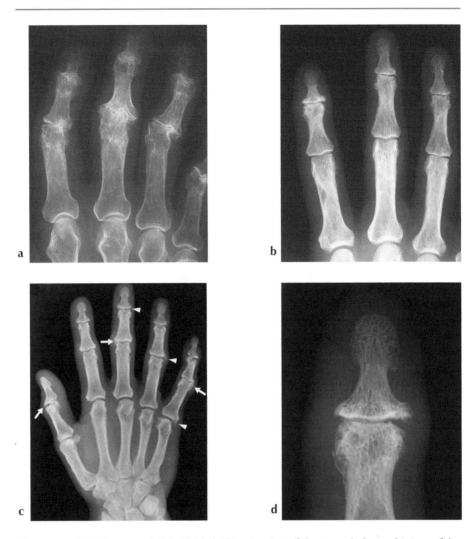

Figure 3.2 Hand osteoarthritis (OA). (a) Erosive OA of the interphalangeal joints of the hand. Severe diffuse loss of joint space, malalignment and osteophytosis is visualized. Note sea-gull sign and malalignment. Additional diffuse osteopenia is present. (b) Early OA of the distal interphalangeal joints. Mild focal joint-space narrowing and osteophytosis are present. (c) Distal and proximal interphalangeal OA. Note osteophytosis (arrows), loose bodies (arrowheads) and joint-space narrowing. Beginning of seagull deformity at the proximal interphalangeal joint of digitum III. Additional OA of the base of the thumb and carpometacarpal joint of digitum I. (d) Magnification radiograph of the distal interphalangeal joint of digitum II. Subchondral sclerosis and mild osteophytosis are present

3.2), as well as in the sacroiliac (SC) joints, where more diffuse joint-space narrowing may be apparent.

Due to the inability of radiography to visualize cartilage directly, cartilage loss must be assessed indirectly from the narrowing of the distance between opposing articular surfaces. However, even small changes in the positioning of the patient can result in large differences in the projection of this space;[14] this is especially relevant if joint-space narrowing is used as a marker of disease progression.[15]

For radiographic assessment of hip joint-space width, computer-assisted methods appear to offer superior precision over manual measurements.[16,17]

Subchondral sclerosis

Usually, subchondral sclerosis detectable with conventional radiography does not develop until cartilage thinning (or loss of articular space) is present. After cartilage loss, the subchondral bone responds with hypervascularization and deposition of new bone on existing trabeculae. Trabecular microfractures and bony collapse with subsequent callus formation may evolve.[18–20] The radioopaque sclerotic areas initially appear uniform but, over time, radiolucent areas representing subchondral cysts may develop within the sclerotic areas.

Subchondral cysts

Cysts are a typical finding in OA, and are known by a multitude of names, including synovial cysts, subchondral cysts or geodes. However, as these cavities are not lined by epithelium, the term pseudocyst is more correct. On radiographic examinations, cysts appear in association with joint-space narrowing and subchondral sclerosis. Two theories are favoured with regard to the pathogenesis of formation of cystic lesions – synovial fluid intrusion and bony contusion. The first theory suggests that elevated intra-articular pressure may lead to the intrusion of joint fluid into the subchondral bone via fissured or ulcerated cartilage. Consequently trabecular resorption may evolve and will eventually lead to cavitation (Figure 3.3). The importance of synovial fluid intrusion in the pathogenesis of subchondral cysts has been supported by recent studies.[21,22] The bony contusion theory postulates that subchondral cysts are a consequence of traumatic bone necrosis following violent impact of two opposing articular surfaces not covered by cartilage. The formation of cystic cavities is a secondary event that occurs during healing and remodelling. This is supported by the often absent communication between the articular cavity and the subchondral cyst. Later investigations have demonstrated that both mechanisms are part of cyst formation in OA.[23]

Characteristically, the cysts observed on radiographic evaluation have a sclerotic margin, and occur in areas of increased joint stress. These cysts are usually multiple and of varying size, rarely exceeding 20 mm (Figure 3.3).[24]

Osteophytosis

It has been suggested that osteophytes evolve as the result of the penetration of blood vessels into the basal layers of remaining intact cartilage, and are a reparative response by the remaining cartilage. They may also develop from periosteal or synovial tissue. This latter phenomenon is most common in the femoral neck, where it is called 'buttressing' (Figure 3.4).[25,26] Radiographically, a radiodense line of variable thickness is observed along a part of, or the entire, femoral neck.

Osteophytes are formed as an attempt to repair and redistribute abnormal joint loading. Marginal osteophytes present radiographically as lips of new bone formation around the edges of the joint, while central osteophytes lead to a bumpy articular contour. Associated chondral defects are often found with central osteophytosis.[27]

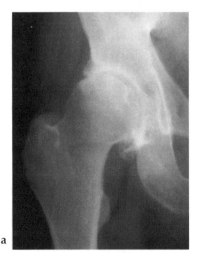 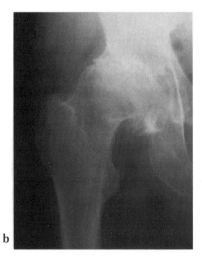

a   b

Figure 3.3 Hip osteoarthritis (OA). (a) and (b) Progressive OA of the hip over a 6-year period. Note progressive cranio-lateral migration of the right femoral head, as well as sclerotic and cystic changes in the acetabulum and femoral head

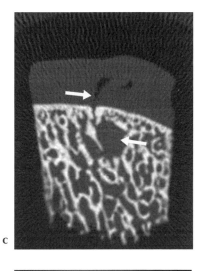

c

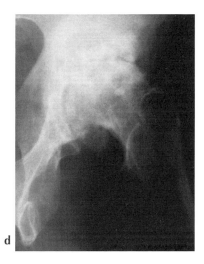

d

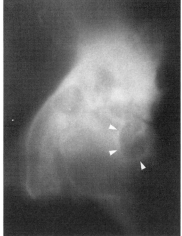

e

Figure 3.3 *continued* (c) Experimental micro-computed tomography imaging (resolution 60 μm) of an osteochondral cylinder depicting an early-stage cyst (arrow). Note cartilage fissure, which is connected via a narrow channel with the subchondral cystic cavity (arrow). (d) Advanced hip OA with marked sclerotic areas and multiform cystic changes. (e) Conventional tomography of a large femoral head cyst. Note marked sclerotic margin of the cyst (arrowheads)

Loose bodies

Intra-articular osteochondral bodies are frequently observed as a complication of OA, particularly in the knee and hip (Figure 3.5a). These bodies may show surface resorption, degenerative calcification or proliferation with deposition of new layers of bone and cartilage.[28] Radiographically, they may change in size, migrate or disappear completely. Joint recesses, such as the fossae of the elbow, the popliteal hiatus of the knee or the axillary pouch and bicipital tendon sheath

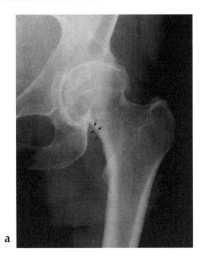
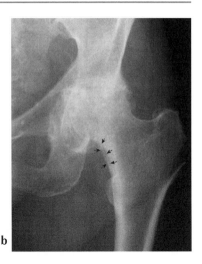

a
b

Figure 3.4 Hip osteoarthritis. Typical examples of femoral neck buttressing seen in patients with osteoarthritis of the hip. The buttress (arrows) can be easily distinguished from the original medial cortex of the femoral neck

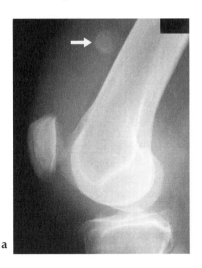
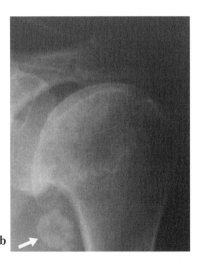

a
b

Figure 3.5 Loose bodies. (a) Lateral radiograph of the knee. An osteochondral body is seen in the patellar pouch of the knee joint (arrow). (b) Anterior–posterior view of the shoulder. Severe osteophytosis of the inferior humeral head and an osteochondral body in the axillary pouch (arrow) are depicted

of the glenohumeral joint, have to be assessed carefully for the presence of loose bodies (Figure 3.5b).[29] It is important to differentiate osteochondral bodies of other origin in such conditions as osteochondritis dissecans or synovial enchondromatosis. Enchondromatosis is a metaplastic condition of synovium associated with a large number of osteocartilaginous bodies of approximately the same size, whereas in OA, only a small number of loose bodies of variable size are usually seen. Osteochondritis dissecans is a condition without features of OA initially, but with the risk of secondary OA during its natural course.

CT and CT-arthrography

CT provides cross-sectional digital images using advanced X-ray technology. A limitation of the technique used to be the transaxial scan orientation, which parallels the joint space of many joints in the body. Since the introduction of helical CT systems, with thin or overlapping sections, this problem has been solved and, if isotropic voxels are acquired, multiplanar reconstructions of any given plane are possible with equal quality to the original plane (Figures 3.6 and 3.7). In comparison with MRI, CT is superior in the visualization of cortical bone and soft-tissue calcifications.

CT and CT-myelography are valuable but increasingly less used techniques for the evaluation of degenerative disc disease, spinal canal stenosis and facet joint OA (Figure 3.6).[30,31] In the peripheral joints, CT has a high sensitivity in the detection of intra-articular loose bony fragments.[32,33]

With the advent of the newer helical multidetector CT systems, a renaissance of CT-arthrography may evolve as an additional tool for initial assessment, as well as for evaluation of the progression of larger osteoarthritic joints. This is particularly true where access to MR facilities is limited or an MR examination is contraindicated. As cartilage is a non-radioopaque structure, its direct visualization by CT or X-ray technology is not possible. However, it has been shown that spiral CT-arthrography of the knee and shoulder is outstanding for imaging the articular surface.[34–37] Penetration of contrast medium (CM) within the cartilage substance indicates a defect of the normally continuous surface. An excellent conspicuity of focal morphologic changes can be achieved, due to the high spatial resolution and high attenuation difference between the cartilage substance and the contrast medium within the joint. A limitation is the insensitivity to changes in the deep layers of cartilage without surface alterations. Qualitative assessment of the knee cartilage using CT-arthrography is comparable to MRI.[35,37,38] Calculation of cartilage volume using CT-arthrography has been performed on human cadaver knees.[39,40]

In summary, CT is a valuable tool for the diagnosis of OA, especially when imaging of osseous changes or detailed pre-surgical planning is required.

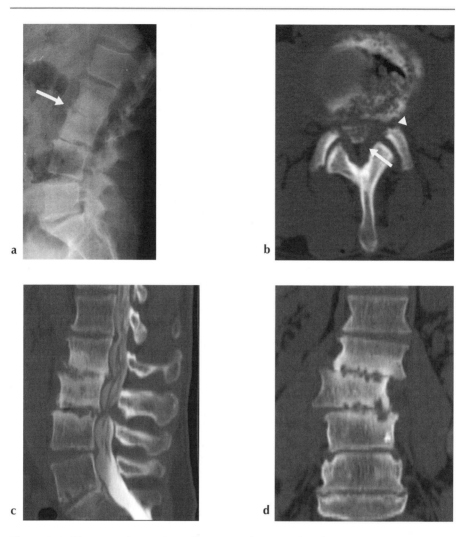

Figure 3.6 Degenerative spine disease with osteochondrosis, apophyseal joint osteoarthritis and spondylosis deformans. Different imaging modalities performed on the same patient prior to surgical intervention. (a) Lateral radiograph. Note diffuse degenerative disc disease of the lumbar spine with complete disc-space obliteration at L2/3 (arrow). (b)–(d) Post-myelographic computed tomography (CT). (b) Axial post-myelographic CT of the intervertebral space at L3/L4. Image shows ligamentum flavum thickening (arrow) and facet hypertrophy with moderate spinal canal stenosis and mild left neural foramen stenosis (arrowhead). (c) Sagittal reformat of the same CT examination. Mild retrolisthesis of L2 to L3 and L3 to L4 is depicted. In comparison with magnetic resonance imaging (MRI) (Figures 3.4e and 3.4f.), CT depicts superiorly disc-space narrowing, bony sclerosis and osteophytosis. (d) Coronal reformat of the same CT examination. Lateral subluxation of L3 towards the right is visualized

(continued overleaf)

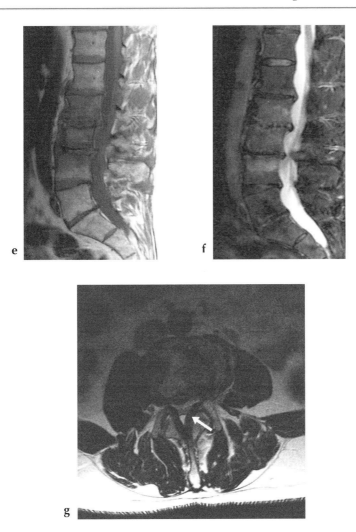

Figure 3.6 *continued* (e)–(g) Non-contrast-enhanced MRI. (e) and (f) Sagittal MRI (T1-weighted and T2-weighted, fat-suppressed sequences). Endplate changes of modic type I (at level L3/4) and type II (at level L4/5) are seen, the former representing oedema and an inflammatory aspect and the latter showing fatty degeneration. (g) Axial T2-weighted MRI at level L3/L4. In comparison with the CT examination, soft tissue is superiorly delineated by MRI. Note hypertrophic ligamentum flavum (arrow)

Drawbacks of CT are low soft-tissue contrast and exposure of the patient to ionizing radiation. CT-arthrography is an alternative imaging method for indirect visualization of cartilage and other intrinsic joint structures, especially in the knee joint.

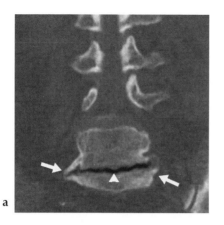
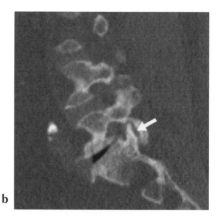

a   b

Figure 3.7 Computed tomography (CT) of degenerative spine disease. (a) Reformatted coronal CT. Image shows vacuum phenomenon in the intervertebral space (arrowhead) and lateral osteophytosis (arrows). (b) Reformatted sagittal CT. A degenerative apophyseal joint with sclerosis, hypertrophy and joint-space narrowing is shown (arrow). Note mild foraminal stenosis

MRI

MRI is based on the natural magnetic behaviour of atomic nuclei within a magnetic field as they spin about their axes. With regard to the physical principles of MRI, we refer the interested reader to the extensive literature available on the topic.[41–43] Although well capable of detecting early changes in OA, MRI is seldom used in routine assessment or initial diagnosis. In comparison with radiography, MRI offers a number of advantages for the imaging of OA. MRI has a tomographic viewing perspective, and thus provides cross-sectional images of the anatomy free of the limitations of radiography. Moreover, MRI is uniquely able to depict directly all components of the joint, including the articular cartilage, menisci, intra-articular ligaments, synovium, capsular structures, bone contours and bone marrow. This allows the joint to be evaluated as a whole organ, and provides a much more detailed picture of the changes associated with OA than is possible with other techniques.[7,44,45]

MRI of cartilage

MRI has emerged as the imaging method of choice for cartilage assessment. Unfortunately, to date, no consensus exists on which of the various imaging sequences is the best for visualization of cartilage. Some of the problems inherent to cartilage imaging, and the currently used sequences, are discussed in this section. Furthermore, an outlook on newer imaging techniques is presented.

T1-weighted conventional spin-echo images offer excellent anatomic detail and high contrast between cartilage and subchondral bone;[46–48] however, they provide insufficient contrast between cartilage, joint fluid and fat, and do not sensitively allow for detection of surface irregularities and focal defects.[46,49] When fat saturation is applied, the grey scale of the T1-weighted image is reset and hyaline cartilage appears as a brighter structure, compared with the adjacent tissues or synovial fluid. Fat suppression also eliminates chemical-shift artefacts (Figure 3.8).[50–53]

The combination of fat suppression with a T1-weighted, three-dimensional gradient-echo technique allows the acquisition of thin slices with high contrast between cartilage and surrounding tissues, and can be reformatted in multiple planes. Signal within cartilage is uniform, and articular cartilage defects can be visualized as contour defects rather than areas of signal change.[51,52,54,55]

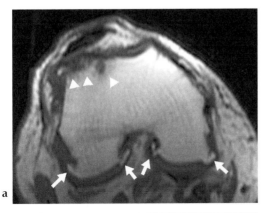

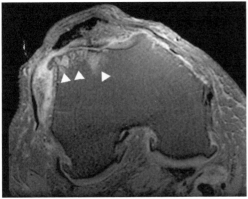

Figure 3.8 Commonly used magnetic resonance pulse sequences for imaging of osteoarthritis. Examples of the same knee. (a) Axial T1-weighted spin-echo sequence. Osseous anatomy is well depicted. Note dorsal femoral osteophytes (arrows). Sub-articular cystic lesions medial and anteriorly appear as low signal areas (arrowheads). (b) Axial T2-weighted spin-echo sequence with fat suppression. In comparison, the cystic changes are delineated superiorly (arrowheads).

(Continued overleaf)

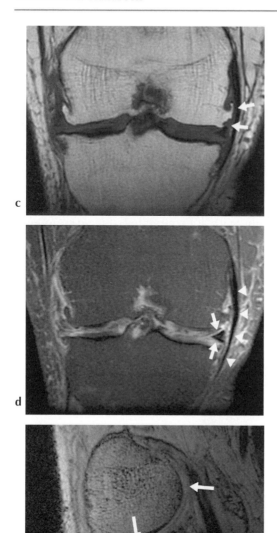

Figure 3.8 *continued* (c) Coronal T2-weighted spin-echo sequence without fat suppression. Excellent visualization of lateral osteophytes (arrows). (d) Coronal T2-weighted sequence with fat suppression. Superior delineation of meniscus (arrows) and collateral ligament (arrowheads) due to fat suppression. (e) Sagittal T2-weighted gradient-echo sequence without fat suppression. Cartilage is depicted as a high signal structure (arrows)

Drawbacks of this technique are the relatively long acquisition time and its susceptibility to metallic artefacts. Using fast spoiled gradient-echo sequences, similar contrast and resolution may be achieved in approximately half the time of the conventional spoiled gradient-echo technique (Figure 3.9).[56] Selective water excitation instead of fat suppression may offer similar time savings.[57,58]

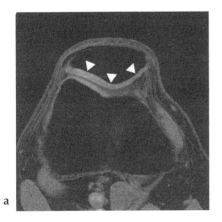
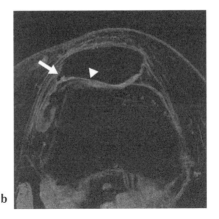

a   b

Figure 3.9 Cartilage imaging by magnetic resonance imaging (MRI). Axial fat-suppressed, T1-weighted, three-dimensional, gradient-echo images of the knee. Cartilage is visualized with high contrast and high spatial resolution. (a) Normal retropatellar cartilage (arrowheads). (b) Thinning of the lateral aspect of the retropatellar cartilage (arrowhead). Note small lateral osteophyte (arrow)

T2-weighted conventional spin-echo imaging offers an arthrogram-like effect of cartilage appearing dark and surrounding tissues, especially joint fluid, being brighter. However, T2-weighted spin-echo techniques have been found to be relatively insensitive in the detection of cartilage defects,[48,51,54] and offer lower spatial resolution (Figure 3.8).

Fast spin-echo imaging allows improved efficiency in image acquisition, with increased signal-to-noise ratio and spatial resolution and decreased acquisition time and motion artefacts. Magnetization transfer effects further improve contrast.[59–61] Proton-density-weighted fast imaging techniques, with and without fat suppression, have equally proved to be sensitive for cartilage imaging.[62,63]

All the sequences described above are routinely available on clinical MR systems and are easy to use.

New techniques for cartilage imaging with MRI are emerging, to non-invasively assess the compositional matrix integrity of cartilage; these include diffusion-weighted MR imaging,[64,65] sequences using ultra-short echo times,[66] magnetization transfer imaging[67–70] and ^{23}Na-MRI.[71–73]

Delayed gadolinium (Gd)-enhanced MRI of cartilage may provide further insight into the matrix integrity of cartilage.[74–76] This method measures the distribution of a negatively charged contrast agent such as Gd-DTPA, which will distribute into the degraded cartilage, and is not repelled by the negatively charged glycosaminoglycans. This technique may allow assessment of the morphologic and biochemical state of cartilage. Ongoing studies will explore its utility in monitoring therapeutic efficacy and disease progression in OA. Due to the higher signal-to-noise ratio, high-field MRI with field strengths of 3 Tesla will be another fascinating tool for the visualization of early structural alterations.[77,78]

Although none of these techniques is presently in routine clinical use, emerging data provide promise that the future will see patient-specific biochemical analysis of cartilage. However, all of these approaches still have to be validated and, at present, are not applicable to the clinical routine.[7]

Quantitative image processing and analysis have an important role in the longitudinal evaluation of cartilage loss and in monitoring response to therapy.[79–82] Most studies have measured global cartilage volume rather than a cartilage defect in isolation.[82,83] With these techniques, cartilage is segmented from the surrounding tissues using a signal-intensity-based thresholding technique applied to a cartilage-sensitive MR sequence.[79] The present techniques of quantification are labour intensive, and it may take an experienced reader up to an hour to quantify cartilage in a single knee; further developments in reducing the time and effort required are necessary before becoming clinically applicable.[7]

Osseous changes

Ill-defined areas of high signal intensity on T2-weighted or short tau inversion recovery images are commonly seen in the subchondral bone in OA (Figure 3.10). On T1-weighted images these alterations appear as areas of non-homogeneous low signal. These changes are often termed bone marrow oedema. However, a recent radiologic–pathologic correlation study in osteoarthritic knees proved that these areas of intraosseous signal change represent a number of non-specific histologic abnormalities that include bone marrow necrosis, bone marrow fibrosis and trabecular abnormalities. Oedema was actually not a major constituent of the MRI abnormalities in such knees.[84] Marrow oedema-like changes are often associated with acute trauma, but these changes sometimes persist and are found years after trauma, probably representing early degenerative post-traumatic alterations.[85,86]

Suggesting a clinical significance of these MRI findings for OA, Felson *et al.* showed a strong association between bone marrow lesions on MRI and the presence of pain in knee OA.[87] Bone marrow oedema-like changes can alter

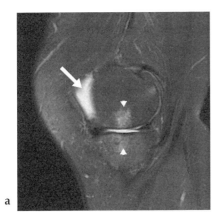
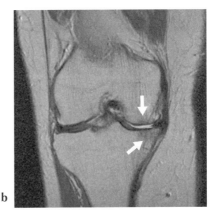

a   b

Figure 3.10 Bone marrow oedema-like changes in osteoarthritis visualized by magnetic resonance imaging (MRI). (a) Sagittal fat-suppressed, T2-weighted image. A subchondral zone of non-homogeneous hyperintensity representing bone marrow oedema-like changes can be seen in the medial femoral condyle and the medial tibial plateau (arrowheads). Note high-signal joint effusion anteriorly (arrow). (b) Coronal T1-weighted image. Areas of non-homogeneous low signal are shown (arrows)

rapidly and it is unknown if interventions that decrease such osseous alterations may also influence pain and/or structural progression.[7]

Other structures including soft tissues

Despite imaging the cartilaginous and osseous structures of a joint, MRI is capable of depicting the intrinsic and surrounding soft tissues,[88] including menisci,[89–92] ligaments,[93] muscles, joint fluid and synovium.[94] Synovitis accompanying OA can be detected by MRI.[95] The usefulness of MRI for evaluation of the glenohumeral ligaments and rotator cuff tears in the shoulder is now well established, as it was previously for the knee.[96–99]

In summary, MRI is superiorly able to visualize directly articular cartilage and soft-tissue changes associated with OA. It has a very high sensitivity for early changes, and quantification of subtle morphological variations in the different articular tissues is possible. MRI may provide more objective measures of disease progression and treatment response than are currently available by other imaging methods. The drawbacks are the relatively long examination time and high costs.

Ultrasonography

Clinical ultrasonography utilizes sound waves of frequencies between 2 and 20 MHz to create images of the human body. In comparison with abdominal ultrasonography, most structures evaluated by musculoskeletal ultrasound are superficial, and therefore, higher-frequency probes are used (10 MHz or more), which support better image quality.

Ultrasound is an effective additional imaging tool in the assessment of OA. This imaging modality is inexpensive, widely available and does not expose the patient to radiation. Joint effusions can be clearly visualized.[100,101] Several studies have also shown loss of joint space,[102] Baker's cysts[103,104] and meniscal abnormalities.[105] Synovitis, as a possible inflammatory component of the disease, may be depicted by sonography even though differentiation of synovitis and joint fluid may be difficult, even with colour or power Doppler.[106,107] The value of ultrasound for the assessment of full-thickness rotator cuff tears of the shoulder, which are often an accompanying feature of OA, is well established, with a sensitivity of 57–100% and specificity of 50–100%.[96,108,109] The potential of ultrasound for the evaluation of calcific tendonitis,[110] acromioclavicular (AC) joint disease,[111] the long head of biceps tendon subluxation, as well as impingement and coracoacromial arch bursitis,[112] remains to be determined.

Ultrasound has also been used for evaluation of the articular cartilage. Normal articular cartilage is seen as a hypoechoic band with sharp margins.[113] An experimental study assessing bovine articular cartilage using high-frequency ultrasonography proved the usefulness of the method for evaluation of the quality of superficial articular cartilage, as well as for measurement of cartilage thickness.[114] In routine clinical practice, cartilage assessment is limited, due mainly to inaccessibility, a result of the small acoustic windows obtainable in most patients. Further drawbacks of the method are its inability to pass through bone and its limitations in evaluation of intra-articular elements, such as the menisci and cruciate ligaments of the knee. This imaging technique is very user-dependent and has limited reproducibility.

Scintigraphy

Scintigraphy uses injectable radiopharmaceuticals to investigate skeletal metabolism, localize disease and contribute to the assessment of the severity of pathologic changes in OA.

Radionuclide scanning with the commonly used radionuclide technetium 99m-hydroxymethylpyrimidine (^{99m}Tc-HDP) reveals increased activity during the bone phase in the subchondral region of the affected joint in nodal OA of the hands.[115] This may even be apparent long before the typical radiographic changes appear, and reflects the vascular reaction and osteoblastic activity present even in the early stages of cartilage loss.

A recent study compared MRI with radionuclide scanning in patients with chronic knee pain. Good agreement was found between increased bone uptake and MR-detected subchondral bone marrow oedema-like lesions, but the agreement between increased bone uptake and osteophytes or cartilage defects was, in general, poor.[116] In another prospective study, scintigraphy proved to be a good predictor for disease progression in knee OA. A normal bone scan at baseline was highly predictive for a lack of progression over a 5-year period.[117] If these data are confirmed, normal scintigraphy at baseline might be very helpful as an exclusion criterion in controlled clinical trials of disease-modifying drugs.

In summary, scintigraphy may be a valuable additional tool in the assessment of OA as it has excellent sensitivity, may demonstrate pathology prior to radiologic changes, and is inexpensive and readily available. The drawback of the technique for the assessment of OA is, primarily, its poor specificity.[118] Currently, bone scintigraphy is rarely used in the diagnosis of OA.

Characteristic imaging features at specific locations

Hands

OA of the hands is common. Typically affected are the distal interphalangeal, proximal interphalangeal and first carpometacarpal joints. In general, involvement is symmetrical and multiple joints are affected. The hallmarks of hand OA are the Heberden's (distal interphalangeal joints) and Bouchard's (proximal interphalangeal joints) nodes. OA of the hands and wrists exhibits the typical radiographic features of the disease, such as osteophytosis and joint-space narrowing. Although joint-space loss is usually focal in OA, in the small interphalangeal joints it may be more diffuse. The undulating contour of the base of the distal phalanx in such a joint creates the so-called 'seagull-sign'. The typical clinical and radiographic characteristics are sufficient for diagnosis in most cases (Figure 3.2).

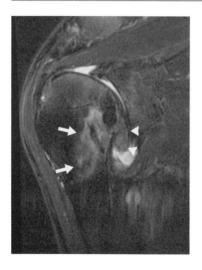

Figure 3.11 Magnetic resonance imaging (MRI) of glenohumeral-joint osteoarthritis (T2-weighted, paracoronal, fat-suppressed image). Joint-space narrowing, effusion and osteophytosis (arrowheads) of the inferior humeral head are well depicted. Note bone marrow oedema-like change in the humeral head and proximal humerus (arrows)

AC joint, shoulder and elbow

Degenerative changes of the AC joint are found regularly in the elderly. Radiographic examination reveals the typical features of OA, plus additional hypertrophy and possible inferior subluxation of the acromial end of the clavicle.

In comparison with degenerative changes in the AC joint, OA of the gleno-humeral and elbow joint is rarely observed in the absence of prior trauma. The most common pathology accompanying OA of the glenohumeral joint is osteophytes along the articular margin of the humeral head and along the site of attachment of the glenoid labrum to the glenoid fossa (Figures 3.5b and 3.11). An associated feature of glenohumeral OA is degeneration of the rotator cuff. It is still unclear if these two conditions are independent phenomena or if a patho-genetic association exists.[24] Measurements of the subacromial space using conventional radiography for the assessment of cuff disease are rarely precise, as the estimates will vary according to the angulation of the X-ray source. Ideal visualization of the subacromial space is achieved with 15–20° caudal angulation of the beam. Further indirect radiographic signs of rotator cuff disease include subacromial osteophytes and defects in the humeral surface near the bicipital groove.

The methods of choice for evaluation of the rotator cuff are MRI and MR-arthrography.[96,119–121]

A special form of atrophic shoulder OA observed in the elderly has been termed the 'Milwaukee shoulder', a result of abnormal accumulation of calcium hydroxyapatite crystals.[122–124]

For complete evaluation of the glenohumeral joint, including secondary soft-tissue changes, MRI or MR-arthrography is required. This may be important prior to surgical intervention. Ultrasound has an important additional role in the assessment of the rotator cuff and possible joint effusions. Plain radiography is almost always required for complete evaluation of the osseous structures, while, at present, CT has only a minor role in shoulder assessment.

Hip

OA of the hip is very common. Taking into account the predominant areas of cartilage loss and subsequent joint-space loss, three patterns can be differentiated. Latero-cranial migration of the femoral head is the type most often observed, presenting unilaterally in most patients.[125] Medio-caudal migration is usually bilateral, and is more common in women.[126] Subchondral sclerosis and cyst formation, as well as joint-space narrowing, are confined to the medial third of the joint. The third axial pattern of migration is infrequent and characterized by concentric diffuse loss of cartilage.[127] In contrast to rheumatoid arthritis, periarticular demineralization is usually missing.

The basic radiographic and pathologic abnormalities are similar for all three migration patterns, i.e. joint-space narrowing, cyst formation, osteophytosis and sclerosis. Cysts, especially in the acetabulum, may be large (Figures 3.3 and 3.12).[128]

Additional MRI or MR-arthrography is helpful in evaluating labral or chondral pathology in detail.[129,130] Indications for MR are unclear joint pain without obvious changes on conventional X-rays, mismatch between clinical findings and radiographic imaging, and before arthroscopic surgery.[131]

Knee

OA of the knee affects a significant percentage of the adult population, resulting in severe degradation of quality of life. The medial tibiofemoral compartment is the site most commonly affected by OA; however, combined medial and lateral changes may also be observed.[118] Joint-space narrowing, osteophyte formation, including central osteophytes, and subchondral sclerosis are seen regularly. Subchondral cysts are small and less common than in the hip.

The patellofemoral compartment is often affected; usually, this involvement is combined with OA changes in the other compartments. An axial view of the patella should be included to evaluate the patellofemoral joint in patients with

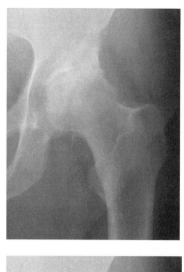

a

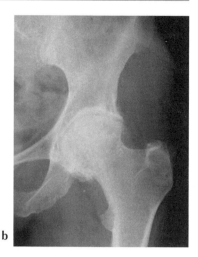

b

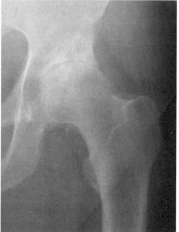

c

Figure 3.12 Patterns of migration in osteoarthritis (OA) of the hip joint. (a) Antero-cranial migration. Note narrowing of the joint space, subchondral cysts and sclerosis. (b) Medio-caudal hip OA. Predominantly medial osteophytosis and joint-space narrowing are found. (c) Axial pattern of migration. Concentric narrowing of the joint space. Little osteophyte formation is observed

suspected knee OA. Patellar subluxation may be evident. Joint effusions are generally small in OA of the knee.

A limitation of routine radiography is its insensitivity in detecting early changes.[118] Additional special radiographic views may be necessary for complete disease assessment and treatment planning. These are weight-bearing views,[132] skyline views, long-leg films, tunnel views[133,134] and stress views.[135] To discuss these techniques in detail goes beyond the scope of this chapter, but extensive reviews on radiography in OA of the knee have been published.[136,137] MRI may provide detailed additional information and is the method of choice for early detection and surveillance of disease progression.

Foot and ankle

OA of the first MTP joint (hallux rigidus and hallux valgus) is very common.[138,139] A predisposing event is usually present in OA of the ankle joint. Most often it appears as a late sequelae after a fracture of the adjacent bones. Radiographic changes observed are osteophytosis, joint-space narrowing, valgus deformity and sclerosis (Figure 3.13).

Spine and sacroiliac joints

The term degenerative disease of the spine is applied to a variety of different processes affecting the various spinal joints. Characteristic degenerative changes are found in each of these joints, including the intervertebral space, the apophyseal or facet joints or the uncovertebral joints of the cervical spine.

Degenerative disc changes are universal. The primary changes are dehydration, fibrous-tissue accumulation and collapse. For detection of the early changes of disc degeneration, MRI is the modality of choice. The degenerative disc shows lower signal intensity on T1- and T2-weighted images. On conventional radiographs or CT images, radiolucent areas (called 'vacuum phenomenon') may be seen, representing gas, mainly nitrogen (Figure 3.7).[140]

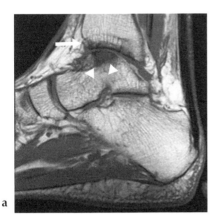 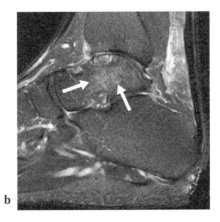

a b

Figure 3.13 Magnetic resonance imaging (MRI) of post-traumatic ankle osteoarthritis. (a) Sagittal T1-weighted image. Marked loss of joint space in the tibiotalar joint with low signal intensity subchondral cystic changes (arrowheads) is shown. Note mild osteophytosis of the anterior tibia (arrow). (b) T2-weighted fat-suppressed image. Additionally, high-signal abnormalities can be seen in the subchondral bone of the talus, representing bone marrow oedema-like changes (arrows)

Disc-space loss and sclerosis are present with more advanced osteochondrosis. Concomitant reactive end-plate signal changes on MRI are observed. Three groups can be differentiated, with type I representing inflammation (Figure 3.6e and f), type II fatty transformation (Figure 3.6e and f) and type III reactive bony replacement.[141,142]

Any segment of the spine may be affected by spinal osteophytosis, called spondylosis deformans.

The apophyseal joints are a common site of OA. The pathologic and radiographic changes are similar to those occurring in other synovial joints. Characteristically, asymmetrical narrowing of the joint space, often in combination with osseous hypertrophy, is observed. Large-facet osteophytes will cause spinal and foraminal stenosis. Optimal visualization of the facet joints requires CT (Figure 3.7).[143] Subluxation may develop in the more advanced stages, which may lead to secondary spondylolisthesis in older patients without a history of spondylolysis, especially at the L4/L5 level, and may be a cause of spinal stenosis.

Although not easily identified radiographically, the sacroiliac joints are a common site of OA. To differentiate these lesions from ankylosing spondylitis may be difficult, but in ankylosing spondylitis, erosions and intra-articular osseous ankylosis are common, while these are infrequent abnormalities in OA. Joint-space narrowing in OA is usually focal.[24]

All imaging methods contribute to the complete assessment of spinal degenerative disease. Depending on the clinical syndrome and therapeutic approach, radiography may be sufficient in some cases. For more detailed analysis, CT, CT-myelography or MRI will be necessary.

Differential diagnosis of osteoarthritis

Taking into account a detailed clinical history and examination plus additional radiographic imaging, the diagnosis of OA is usually straightforward. The following entities have to be considered in the differential diagnosis.

In rheumatoid arthritis, more marked joint effusions, osteoporosis and uniform joint-space loss are present. Bony sclerosis and osteophytosis are not prominent features of rheumatoid arthritis.

Calcium pyrophosphate dihydrate deposition disease shows very similar findings to OA. However, typical intra- and extra-articular calcification of soft tissues and cartilage is not a common feature of OA (Figure 3.14).

Subluxations, malalignment, large effusions, fragmentation and collapse of the articular surfaces characterize the findings in neuropathic osteoarthropathy. Multiple loose bodies may be found.

Preserved joint-space width in combination with focal collapse of subchondral bone is characteristic of osteonecrosis. However, evolving secondary degenerative changes may not be distinguished from so-called primary OA.

Further rare diseases of joints may lead to secondary degenerative changes that will resemble idiopathic OA, such as osteochondritis dissecans, acromegaly, haemophilia, haemochromatosis, Paget's disease or alkaptonuria.

Inflammatory or erosive OA of the hands may be confused with other erosive arthropathies. The characteristic symmetrical distal interphalangeal distribution and predominance of central rather than marginal changes will lead to the diagnosis of OA (Figure 3.2). In distinguishing erosive OA from psoriatic arthritis, the latter condition is characterized by marginal erosions and poorly defined bony proliferations. Psoriatic changes may be distributed asymmetrically, unilaterally or ray-like.[144]

SERUM AND MOLECULAR MARKERS

All imaging modalities provide a historical view of changes that have already occurred, rather than assessing the rate of current disease progression. Molecular markers may help in the diagnosis of disease as well as monitoring progression.

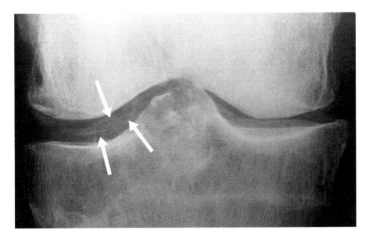

Figure 3.14 Differential diagnosis of osteoarthritis. Calcium pyrophosphate dihydrate deposition disease of the knee joint. Note pathognomonic chondrocalcinosis (arrows)

A good marker should be disease-specific and sensitive to therapy, and should reflect actual disease activity as well as predict disease outcome.

At present, there is no reliable diagnostic test for OA. Analysis of synovial fluid shows non-specific features, such as increased volume, decreased viscosity, mild pleocytosis and a slight decrease in synovial fluid protein – all signs of mild inflammation.

A biochemical marker that accurately reflects the changes in articular cartilage in OA has not yet been identified. Candidate markers for cartilage turnover in OA include molecules present during cartilage matrix synthesis and degradation, such as type II collagen degradation and synthesis (c-propeptide) markers, cartilage oligomeric protein, as well as two epitopes of aggrecan.[145,146] The role of synovial fluid components, serum levels of insulin-like growth factor and urinary excretion of collagen cross-link proteins remains to be determined.[147–150]

The markers that have been examined can be grouped into five clusters (inflammation markers, bone markers, cartilage synthesis markers, cartilage degradation markers and transforming growth factor-β), but none of them can successfully distinguish OA patients from control subjects.[151,152] The future will show if a combination of multiple markers will increase disease specificity and reduce the overlap in individual marker levels that exists between OA patients and control subjects.[153] Currently, laboratory tests in routine clinical practice are used to help exclude other joint disorders from the differential diagnosis.

CONCLUSIONS

Conventional radiography combined with clinical examination remains the first-line diagnostic method for everyday assessment and initial diagnosis of OA. The clinician must determine what the objectives are before more advanced imaging is undertaken. MRI and CT, as well as ultrasound, may add to the complete evaluation of an osteoarthritic joint. MRI in particular has a vital role in clinical and therapeutic trials, and is capable of depicting early changes as well as mild disease progression. With CT, excellent visualization of osseous structures is provided, while ultrasound is primarily used for the assessment of the surrounding soft tissues of a joint. At present, scintigraphic methods as well as laboratory tests have only a minor role in the diagnosis of OA.

References

1. Ehrlich GE. Inflammatory osteoarthritis. I. The clinical syndrome. J Chronic Dis 1972; 25: 317–28

2. Ike R, O'Rourke KS. Compartment-directed physical examination of the knee can predict articular cartilage abnormalities disclosed by needle arthroscopy. Arthritis Rheum 1995; 38: 917–25

3. Altman R, Asch E, Bloch D, et al. Development of criteria for the classification and reporting of osteoarthritis. Classification of osteoarthritis of the knee. Diagnostic and Therapeutic Criteria Committee of the American Rheumatism Association. Arthritis Rheum 1986; 29: 1039–49

4. Altman R, Alarcon G, Appelrouth D, et al. The American College of Rheumatology criteria for the classification and reporting of osteoarthritis of the hand. Arthritis Rheum 1990; 33: 1601–10

5. Altman R, Alarcon G, Appelrouth D, et al. The American College of Rheumatology criteria for the classification and reporting of osteoarthritis of the hip. Arthritis Rheum 1991; 34: 505–14

6. Dieppe P, Peterfy CG, Watt I. Osteoarthritis and related disorders: imaging. In Klippel JH, Dieppe P, eds. Rheumatology, 2nd edn. London: Mosby, 1998: 8.4.1–8.4.10

7. Peterfy CG. Imaging of the disease process. Curr Opin Rheumatol 2002; 14: 590–6

8. Buckland-Wright JC, Wolfe F, Ward RJ, et al. Substantial superiority of semi-flexed (MTP) views in knee osteoarthritis: a comparative radiographic study, without fluoroscopy, of standing extended, semiflexed (MTP), and schuss views. J Rheumatol 1999; 26: 2664–74

9. Mazzuca SA, Brandt KD, Buckwalter KA, et al. Field test of the reproducibility of the semiflexed metatarsophalangeal view in repeated radiographic examinations of subjects with osteoarthritis of the knee. Arthritis Rheum 2002; 46: 109–13

10. Peterfy CG, Li J, Zaim S, et al. Comparison of fixed-flexion positioning with fluoroscopic semi-flexed positioning for quantifying radiographic joint-space width in the knee: test–retest reproducibility. Skeletal Radiol 2003; 32: 128–32

11. Buckland-Wright JC, Macfarlane DG, Jasani MK, Lynch JA. Quantitative microfocal radiographic assessment of osteoarthritis of the knee from weight bearing tunnel and semiflexed standing views. J Rheumatol 1994; 21: 1734–41

12. Mazzuca SA, Brandt KD, Buckland-Wright JC, et al. Field test of the reproducibility of automated measurements of medial tibiofemoral joint space width derived from standardized knee radiographs. J Rheumatol 1999; 26: 1359–65

13. Sharma L, Song J, Felson DT, et al. The role of knee alignment in disease progression and functional decline in knee osteoarthritis. J Am Med Assoc 2001; 286: 188–95

14. Ravaud P, Chastang C, Auleley GR, et al. Assessment of joint space width in patients with osteoarthritis of the knee: a comparison of 4 measuring instruments. J Rheumatol 1996; 23: 1749–55

15. Boegard TL, Rudling O, Petersson IF, Jonsson K. Joint space width of the tibiofemoral and of the patellofemoral joint in chronic knee pain with or without radiographic osteoarthritis: a 2-year follow-up. Osteoarthritis Cartilage 2003; 11: 370–6

16. Conrozier T, Lequesne M, Favret H, et al. Measurement of the radiological hip joint space width. An evaluation of various methods of measurement. Osteoarthritis Cartilage 2001; 9: 281–6

17. Gordon CL, Wu C, Peterfy CG, et al. Automated measurement of radiographic hip joint-space width. Med Phys 2001; 28: 267–77

18. Havdrup T, Hulth A, Telhag H. The subchondral bone in osteoarthritis and rheumatoid arthritis of the knee. A histological and microradiographical study. Acta Orthop Scand 1976; 47: 345–50

19. Kusakabe A. Subchondral cancellous bone in osteoarthrosis and rheumatoid arthritis of the femoral head. A quantitative histological study of trabecular remodelling. Arch Orthop Unfallchir 1977; 88: 185–97

20. Cameron HU, Fornasier VL. Trabecular stress fractures. Clin Orthop 1975: 266–8

21. Schmalzried TP, Akizuki KH, Fedenko AN, Mirra J. The role of access of joint fluid to bone in periarticular osteolysis. A report of four cases. J Bone Joint Surg Am 1997; 79: 447–52

22. Crawford R, Sabokbar A, Wulke A, et al. Expansion of an osteoarthritic cyst associated with wear debris: a case report. J Bone Joint Surg Br 1998; 80: 990–3

23. Resnick D, Niwayama G, Coutts RD. Subchondral cysts (geodes) in arthritic disorders: pathologic and radiographic appearance of the hip joint. Am J Roentgenol 1977; 128: 799–806

24. Resnick D. Degenerative diseases. In Resnick D, ed. Diagnosis of Bone and Joint Disorders, 4th edn. Philadelphia: WB Saunders Company, 2002: 1269–475

25. Martel W, Braunstein EM. The diagnostic value of buttressing of the femoral neck. Arthritis Rheum 1978; 21: 161–4

26. Dixon T, Benjamin J, Lund P, et al. Femoral neck buttressing: a radiographic and histologic analysis. Skeletal Radiol 2000; 29: 587–92

27. McCauley TR, Kornaat PR, Jee WH. Central osteophytes in the knee: prevalence and association with cartilage defects on MR imaging. Am J Roentgenol 2001; 176: 359–64

28. Milgram JW. The development of loose bodies in human joints. Clin Orthop 1977: 292–303

29. Karnahl HM. Unusual stone formation in Baker cysts. Rofo Fortschr Geb Rontgenstr Nuklearmed 1980; 133: 333–5

30. Voelker JL, Mealey J Jr, Eskridge JM, Gilmor RL. Metrizamide-enhanced computed tomography as an adjunct to metrizamide myelography in the evaluation of lumbar disc herniation and spondylosis. Neurosurgery 1987; 20: 379–84

31. Ketonen L, Gyldensted C. Lumbar disc disease evaluated by myelography and postmyelography spinal computed tomography. Neuroradiology 1986; 28: 144–9

32. Brossmann J, Preidler KW, Daenen B, et al. Imaging of osseous and cartilaginous intraarticular bodies in the knee: comparison of MR imaging and MR arthrography with CT and CT arthrography in cadavers. Radiology 1996; 200: 509–17

33. Steinbach LS, Schwartz M. Elbow arthrography. Radiol Clin North Am 1998; 36: 635–49

34. Tuite MJ, Rubin D. CT and MR arthrography of the glenoid labroligamentous complex. Semin Musculoskelet Radiol 1998; 2: 363–76

35. Vande Berg BC, Lecouvet FE, Poilvache P, et al. Assessment of knee cartilage in cadavers with dual-detector spiral CT arthrography and MR imaging. Radiology 2002; 222: 430–6

36. Rand T, Brossmann J, Pedowitz R, et al. Analysis of patellar cartilage. Comparison of conventional MR imaging and MR and CT arthrography in cadavers. Acta Radiol 2000; 41: 492–7

37. Daenen BR, Ferrara MA, Marcelis S, Dondelinger RF. Evaluation of patellar cartilage surface lesions: comparison of CT arthrography and fat-suppressed FLASH 3D MR imaging. Eur Radiol 1998; 8: 981–5

38. Gagliardi JA, Chung EM, Chandnani VP, et al. Detection and staging of chondro-malacia patellae: relative efficacies of conventional MR imaging, MR arthrography, and CT arthrography. Am J Roentgenol 1994; 163: 629–36

39. Schnier M, Eckstein F, Priebsch J, et al. Three-dimensional thickness and volume measurements of the knee joint cartilage using MRI: validation in an anatomical specimen by CT arthrography. Rofo Fortschr Geb Rontgenstr Neuen Bildgeb Verfahr 1997; 167: 521–6

40. Haubner M, Eckstein F, Schnier M, et al. A non-invasive technique for 3-dimensional assessment of articular cartilage thickness based on MRI. Part 2: validation using CT arthrography. Magn Reson Imaging 1997; 15: 805–13

41. Budinger TF, Lauterbur PC. Nuclear magnetic resonance technology for medical studies. Science 1984; 226: 288–98

42. Pykett IL. NMR imaging in medicine. Sci Am 1982; 246: 78–88

43. Elster AD, Burdette J. Questions and Answers in Magnetic Resonance Imaging, 2nd edn. St Louis: Mosby, 2001

44. Peterfy C. Magnetic resonance imaging. In Brandt KD, Doherty M, Lohmander S, eds. Osteoarthritis. New York: Oxford University Press, 1998: 473–94

45. Peterfy CG, Guermazi A, Zaim S, et al. Whole-Organ Magnetic Resonance Imaging Score (WORMS) of the knee in osteoarthritis. Osteoarthritis Cartilage 2004; 12: 177–90

46. Hayes CW, Sawyer RW, Conway WF. Patellar cartilage lesions: in vitro detection and staging with MR imaging and pathologic correlation. Radiology 1990; 176: 479–83

47. Karvonen RL, Negendank WG, Fraser SM, et al. Articular cartilage defects of the knee: correlation between magnetic resonance imaging and gross pathology. Ann Rheum Dis 1990; 49: 672–5

48. Yulish BS, Montanez J, Goodfellow DB, et al. Chondromalacia patellae: assessment with MR imaging. Radiology 1987; 164: 763–6

49. Hayes CW, Conway WF. Evaluation of articular cartilage: radiographic and cross-sectional imaging techniques. Radiographics 1992; 12: 409–28

50. Chandnani VP, Ho C, Chu P, et al. Knee hyaline cartilage evaluated with MR imaging: a cadaveric study involving multiple imaging sequences and intraarticular injection of gadolinium and saline solution. Radiology 1991; 178: 557–61

51. Disler DG, McCauley TR, Kelman CG, et al. Fat-suppressed three-dimensional spoiled gradient-echo MR imaging of hyaline cartilage defects in the knee: comparison with standard MR imaging and arthroscopy. Am J Roentgenol 1996; 167: 127–32

52. Disler DG, McCauley TR, Wirth CR, Fuchs MD. Detection of knee hyaline cartilage defects using fat-suppressed three-dimensional spoiled gradient-echo MR imaging: comparison with standard MR imaging and correlation with arthroscopy. Am J Roentgenol 1995; 165: 377–82

53. Rose PM, Demlow TA, Szumowski J, Quinn SF. Chondromalacia patellae: fat-suppressed MR imaging. Radiology 1994; 193: 437–40

54. Recht MP, Kramer J, Marcelis S, et al. Abnormalities of articular cartilage in the knee: analysis of available MR techniques. Radiology 1993; 187: 473–8

55. Recht MP, Piraino DW, Paletta GA, et al. Accuracy of fat-suppressed three-dimensional spoiled gradient-echo FLASH MR imaging in the detection of patellofemoral articular cartilage abnormalities. Radiology 1996; 198: 209–12

56. Cicuttini F, Forbes A, Asbeutah A, et al. Comparison and reproducibility of fast and conventional spoiled gradient-echo magnetic resonance sequences in the determination of knee cartilage volume. J Orthop Res 2000; 18: 580–4

57. Glaser C, Faber S, Eckstein F, et al. Optimization and validation of a rapid high-resolution T1-w 3D FLASH water excitation MRI sequence for the quantitative assessment of articular cartilage volume and thickness. Magn Reson Imaging 2001; 19: 177–85

58. Mohr A, Priebe M, Taouli B, et al. Selective water excitation for faster MR imaging of articular cartilage defects: initial clinical results. Eur Radiol 2003; 13: 686–9

59. Yao L, Gentili A, Thomas A. Incidental magnetization transfer contrast in fast spin-echo imaging of cartilage. J Magn Reson Imaging 1996; 6: 180–4

60. Potter HG, Linklater JM, Allen AA, et al. Magnetic resonance imaging of articular cartilage in the knee. An evaluation with use of fast-spin-echo imaging. J Bone Joint Surg Am 1998; 80: 1276–84

61. Bredella MA, Tirman PF, Peterfy CG, et al. Accuracy of T2-weighted fast spin-echo MR imaging with fat saturation in detecting cartilage defects in the knee: comparison with arthroscopy in 130 patients. Am J Roentgenol 1999; 172: 1073–80

62. Sonin AH, Pensy RA, Mulligan ME, Hatem S. Grading articular cartilage of the knee using fast spin-echo proton density-weighted MR imaging without fat suppression. Am J Roentgenol 2002; 179: 1159–66

63. Mohr A. The value of water-excitation 3D FLASH and fat-saturated PDw TSE MR imaging for detecting and grading articular cartilage lesions of the knee. Skeletal Radiol 2003; 32: 396–402

64. Burstein D, Gray ML, Hartman AL, et al. Diffusion of small solutes in cartilage as measured by nuclear magnetic resonance (NMR) spectroscopy and imaging. J Orthop Res 1993; 11: 465–78

65. Xia Y, Farquhar T, Burton-Wurster N, et al. Diffusion and relaxation mapping of cartilage-bone plugs and excised disks using microscopic magnetic resonance imaging. Magn Reson Med 1994; 31: 273–82

66. Brossmann J, Frank LR, Pauly JM, et al. Short echo time projection reconstruction MR imaging of cartilage: comparison with fat-suppressed spoiled GRASS and magnetization transfer contrast MR imaging. Radiology 1997; 203: 501–7

67. Wolff SD, Chesnick S, Frank JA, et al. Magnetization transfer contrast: MR imaging of the knee. Radiology 1991; 179: 623–8

68. Kim DK, Ceckler TL, Hascall VC, et al. Analysis of water-macromolecule proton magnetization transfer in articular cartilage. Magn Reson Med 1993; 29: 211–15

69. Hohe J, Faber S, Stammberger T, et al. A technique for 3D in vivo quantification of proton density and magnetization transfer coefficients of knee joint cartilage. Osteoarthritis Cartilage 2000; 8: 426–33

70. Gray ML, Burstein D, Lesperance LM, Gehrke L. Magnetization transfer in cartilage and its constituent macromolecules. Magn Reson Med 1995; 34: 319–25

71. Reddy R, Insko EK, Noyszewski EA, et al. Sodium MRI of human articular cartilage in vivo. Magn Reson Med 1998; 39: 697–701

72. Shapiro EM, Borthakur A, Dandora R, et al. Sodium visibility and quantitation in intact bovine articular cartilage using high field (23)Na MRI and MRS. J Magn Reson 2000; 142: 24–31

73. Shapiro EM, Borthakur A, Gougoutas A, Reddy R. 23Na MRI accurately measures fixed charge density in articular cartilage. Magn Reson Med 2002; 47: 284–91

74. Bashir A, Gray ML, Boutin RD, Burstein D. Glycosaminoglycan in articular cartilage: in vivo assessment with delayed Gd(DTPA)(2-)-enhanced MR imaging. Radiology 1997; 205: 551–8

75. Bashir A, Gray ML, Hartke J, Burstein D. Nondestructive imaging of human cartilage glycosaminoglycan concentration by MRI. Magn Reson Med 1999; 41: 857–65

76. Burstein D, Bashir A, Gray ML. MRI techniques in early stages of cartilage disease. Invest Radiol 2000; 35: 622–38

77. Peterson DM, Carruthers CE, Wolverton BL, et al. Application of a birdcage coil at 3 Tesla to imaging of the human knee using MRI. Magn Reson Med 1999; 42: 215–21

78. Chung CB, Frank LR, Resnick D. Cartilage imaging techniques: current clinical applications and state of the art imaging. Clin Orthop 2001: S370–8

79. Peterfy CG, van Dijke CF, Janzen DL, et al. Quantification of articular cartilage in the knee with pulsed saturation transfer subtraction and fat-suppressed MR imaging: optimization and validation. Radiology 1994; 192: 485–91

80. Peterfy CG, van Dijke CF, Lu Y, et al. Quantification of the volume of articular cartilage in the metacarpophalangeal joints of the hand: accuracy and precision of three-dimensional MR imaging. Am J Roentgenol 1995; 165: 371–5

81. Piplani MA, Disler DG, McCauley TR, et al. Articular cartilage volume in the knee: semiautomated determination from three-dimensional reformations of MR images. Radiology 1996; 198: 855–9

82. Eckstein F, Schnier M, Haubner M, et al. Accuracy of cartilage volume and thickness measurements with magnetic resonance imaging. Clin Orthop 1998: 137–48

83. Losch A, Eckstein F, Haubner M, Englmeier KH. A non-invasive technique for 3-dimensional assessment of articular cartilage thickness based on MRI. Part 1: development of a computational method. Magn Reson Imaging 1997; 15: 795–804

84. Zanetti M, Bruder E, Romero J, Hodler J. Bone marrow oedema pattern in osteoarthritic knees: correlation between MR imaging and histologic findings. Radiology 2000; 215: 835–40

85. Vellet AD, Marks PH, Fowler PJ, Munro TG. Occult posttraumatic osteochondral lesions of the knee: prevalence, classification, and short-term sequelae evaluated with MR imaging. Radiology 1991; 178: 271–6

86. Roemer FW, Bohndorf K. Long-term osseous sequelae after acute trauma of the knee joint evaluated by MRI. Skeletal Radiol 2002; 31: 615–23

87. Felson DT, Chaisson CE, Hill CL, et al. The association of bone marrow lesions with pain in knee osteoarthritis. Ann Intern Med 2001; 134: 541–9

88. Chan WP, Lang P, Stevens MP, et al. Osteoarthritis of the knee: comparison of radiography, CT, and MR imaging to assess extent and severity. Am J Roentgenol 1991; 157: 799–806

89. Reicher MA, Hartzman S, Duckwiler GR, et al. Meniscal injuries: detection using MR imaging. Radiology 1986; 159: 753–7

90. De Smet AA, Norris MA, Yandow DR, et al. Diagnosis of meniscal tears of the knee with MR imaging: effect of observer variation and sample size on sensitivity and specificity. Am J Roentgenol 1993; 160: 555–9

91. De Smet AA, Norris MA, Yandow DR, et al. MR diagnosis of meniscal tears of the knee: importance of high signal in the meniscus that extends to the surface. Am J Roentgenol 1993; 161: 101–7

92. Quinn SF, Brown TR, Szumowski J. Menisci of the knee: radial MR imaging correlated with arthroscopy in 259 patients. Radiology 1992; 185: 577–80

93. Rubin DA, Kettering JM, Towers JD, Britton CA. MR imaging of knees having isolated and combined ligament injuries. Am J Roentgenol 1998; 170: 1207–13

94. Guermazi A, Zaim S, Taouli B, et al. MR findings in knee osteoarthritis. Eur Radiol 2003; 13: 1370–86

95. Fernandez-Madrid F, Karvonen RL, Teitge RA, et al. Synovial thickening detected by MR imaging in osteoarthritis of the knee confirmed by biopsy as synovitis. Magn Reson Imaging 1995; 13: 177–83

96. Kluger R, Mayrhofer R, Kroner A, et al. Sonographic versus magnetic resonance arthrographic evaluation of full-thickness rotator cuff tears in millimeters. J Shoulder Elbow Surg 2003; 12: 110–16

97. Yeh L, Kwak S, Kim YS, et al. Anterior labroligamentous structures of the gleno-humeral joint: correlation of MR arthrography and anatomic dissection in cadav-ers. Am J Roentgenol 1998; 171: 1229–36

98. Stoller DW. MR arthrography of the glenohumeral joint. Radiol Clin North Am 1997; 35: 97–116

99. Steinbach LS, Gunther SB. Magnetic resonance imaging of the rotator cuff. Semin Roentgenol 2000; 35: 200–16

100. Iagnocco A, Coari G. Usefulness of high resolution US in the evaluation of effusion in osteoarthritic first carpometacarpal joint. Scand J Rheumatol 2000; 29: 170–3

101. Bierma-Zeinstra SM, Bohnen AM, Verhaar JA, et al. Sonography for hip joint effusion in adults with hip pain. Ann Rheum Dis 2000; 59: 178–82

102. Iagnocco A, Coari G, Zoppini A. Sonographic evaluation of femoral condylar cartilage in osteoarthritis and rheumatoid arthritis. Scand J Rheumatol 1992; 21: 201–3

103. Helbich TH, Breitenseher M, Trattnig S, et al. Sonomorphologic variants of popliteal cysts. J Clin Ultrasound 1998; 26: 171–6

104. Ward EE, Jacobson JA, Fessell DP, et al. Sonographic detection of Baker's cysts: comparison with MR imaging. Am J Roentgenol 2001; 176: 373–80

105. Rutten MJ, Collins JM, van Kampen A, Jager GJ. Meniscal cysts: detection with high-resolution sonography. Am J Roentgenol 1998; 171: 491–6

106. Newman JS, Laing TJ, McCarthy CJ, Adler RS. Power Doppler sonography of synovitis: assessment of therapeutic response – preliminary observations. Radiology 1996; 198: 582–4

107. Rubin JM. Musculoskeletal power Doppler. Eur Radiol 1999; 9 (Suppl 3): S403–6

108. Swen WA, Jacobs JW, Algra PR, et al. Sonography and magnetic resonance imaging equivalent for the assessment of full-thickness rotator cuff tears. Arthritis Rheum 1999; 42: 2231–8

109. Teefey SA, Middleton WD, Yamaguchi K. Shoulder sonography. State of the art. Radiol Clin North Am 1999; 37: 767–85

110. Farin PU, Rasanen H, Jaroma H, Harju A. Rotator cuff calcifications: treatment with ultrasound-guided percutaneous needle aspiration and lavage. Skeletal Radiol 1996; 25: 551–4

111. Fenkl R, Gotzen L. Sonographic diagnosis of the injured acromioclavicular joint. A standardized examination procedure. Unfallchirurg 1992; 95: 393–400

112. Read JW, Perko M. Shoulder ultrasound: diagnostic accuracy for impingement syndrome, rotator cuff tear, and biceps tendon pathology. J Shoulder Elbow Surg 1998; 7: 264–71

113. Ostergaard M, Court-Payen M, Gideon P, et al. Ultrasonography in arthritis of the knee. A comparison with MR imaging. Acta Radiol 1995; 36: 19–26

114. Toyras J, Nieminen HJ, Laasanen MS, et al. Ultrasonic characterization of articular cartilage. Biorheology 2002; 39: 161–9

115. Hutton CW, Higgs ER, Jackson PC, et al. 99mTc HMDP bone scanning in generalised nodal osteoarthritis. II. The four hour bone scan image predicts radiographic change. Ann Rheum Dis 1986; 45: 622–6

116. Boegard T, Rudling O, Dahlstrom J, et al. Bone scintigraphy in chronic knee pain: comparison with magnetic resonance imaging. Ann Rheum Dis 1999; 58: 20–6

117. Dieppe P, Cushnaghan J, Young P, Kirwan J. Prediction of the progression of joint space narrowing in osteoarthritis of the knee by bone scintigraphy. Ann Rheum Dis 1993; 52: 557–63

118. Thomas RH, Resnick D, Alazraki NP, et al. Compartmental evaluation of osteoarthritis of the knee. A comparative study of available diagnostic modalities. Radiology 1975; 116: 585–94

119. Tirman PF, Bost FW, Steinbach LS, et al. MR arthrographic depiction of tears of the rotator cuff: benefit of abduction and external rotation of the arm. Radiology 1994; 192: 851–6

120. Flannigan B, Kursunoglu-Brahme S, Snyder S, et al. MR arthrography of the shoulder: comparison with conventional MR imaging. Am J Roentgenol 1990; 155: 829–32

121. Palmer WE, Brown JH, Rosenthal DI. Rotator cuff: evaluation with fat-suppressed MR arthrography. Radiology 1993; 188: 683–7

122. Garancis JC, Cheung HS, Halverson PB, McCarty DJ. 'Milwaukee shoulder' – association of microspheroids containing hydroxyapatite crystals, active collagenase, and neutral protease with rotator cuff defects. III. Morphologic and biochemical studies of an excised synovium showing chondromatosis. Arthritis Rheum 1981; 24: 484–91

123. Halverson PB, Cheung HS, McCarty DJ, et al. 'Milwaukee shoulder' – association of microspheroids containing hydroxyapatite crystals, active collagenase, and neutral protease with rotator cuff defects. II. Synovial fluid studies. Arthritis Rheum 1981; 24: 474–83

124. McCarty DJ, Halverson PB, Carrera GF, et al. 'Milwaukee shoulder' – association of microspheroids containing hydroxyapatite crystals, active collagenase, and

neutral protease with rotator cuff defects. I. Clinical aspects. Arthritis Rheum 1981; 24: 464–73

125. Ledingham J, Dawson S, Preston B, et al. Radiographic patterns and associations of osteoarthritis of the hip. Ann Rheum Dis 1992; 51: 1111–16

126. Resnick D. Patterns of migration of the femoral head in osteoarthritis of the hip. Roentgenographic–pathologic correlation and comparison with rheumatoid arthritis. Am J Roentgenol Radium Ther Nucl Med 1975; 124: 62–74

127. Cameron HU, Macnab I. Observations on osteoarthritis of the hip joint. Clin Orthop 1975: 31–40

128. Silas SI, Resnik CS, Levine AM. Bilateral primary cystic arthrosis of the acetabulum. A case report. J Bone Joint Surg Am 1996; 78: 775–8

129. Petersilge CA, Haque MA, Petersilge WJ, et al. Acetabular labral tears: evaluation with MR arthrography. Radiology 1996; 200: 231–5

130. Czerny C, Hofmann S, Neuhold A, et al. Lesions of the acetabular labrum: accuracy of MR imaging and MR arthrography in detection and staging. Radiology 1996; 200: 225–30

131. Imhof H, Czerny C, Gahleitner A, et al. Coxarthrosis. Radiologe 2002; 42: 416–31

132. Leach RE, Gregg T, Siber FJ. Weight-bearing radiography in osteoarthritis of the knee. Radiology 1970; 97: 265–8

133. Resnick D, Vint V. The 'Tunnel' view in assessment of cartilage loss in osteoarthritis of the knee. Radiology 1980; 137: 547–8

134. Marklund T, Myrnerts R. Radiographic determination of cartilage height in the knee joint. Acta Orthop Scand 1974; 45: 752–5

135. Gibson PH, Goodfellow JW. Stress radiography in degenerative arthritis of the knee. J Bone Joint Surg Br 1986; 68: 608–9

136. Boegard T, Jonsson K. Radiography in osteoarthritis of the knee. Skeletal Radiol 1999; 28: 605–15

137. Mazzuca SA, Brandt KD. Plain radiography as an outcome measure in clinical trials involving patients with knee osteoarthritis. Rheum Dis Clin North Am 1999; 25: 467–80

138. Mann RA, Coughlin MJ, DuVries HL. Hallux rigidus: a review of the literature and a method of treatment. Clin Orthop 1979: 57–63

139. Mann RA, Coughlin MJ. Hallux valgus – etiology, anatomy, treatment and surgical considerations. Clin Orthop 1981: 31–41

140. Ford LT, Gilula LA, Murphy WA, Gado M. Analysis of gas in vacuum lumbar disc. Am J Roentgenol 1977; 128: 1056–7

141. Modic MT, Steinberg PM, Ross JS, et al. Degenerative disk disease: assessment of changes in vertebral body marrow with MR imaging. Radiology 1988; 166: 193–9

142. Modic MT, Masaryk TJ, Ross JS, Carter JR. Imaging of degenerative disk disease. Radiology 1988; 168: 177–86

143. Harvey CJ, Richenberg JL, Saifuddin A, Wolman RL. The radiological investigation of lumbar spondylolysis. Clin Radiol 1998; 53: 723–8

144. Martel W, Stuck KJ, Dworin AM, Hylland RG. Erosive osteoarthritis and psoriatic arthritis: a radiologic comparison in the hand, wrist, and foot. Am J Roentgenol 1980; 134: 125–35

145. Thonar EJM, Manicourt DH. Noninvasive markers in osteoarthritis. In Moskowitz RW, Howell DS, Altman RD, et al., eds. Osteoarthritis, 3rd edn. Philadelphia: WB Saunders, 2001: 293–314

146. Poole AR. Can osteoarthritis as a disease be distinguished from ageing by skeletal and inflammation markers? Implications for 'early' diagnosis, monitoring skeletal changes and effects of therapy. In Hamerman D, ed. Osteoarthritis: Public Health Implications for an Aging Population. Baltimore: Johns Hopkins University Press, 1997: 187–214

147. Lohmander LS, Lark MW, Dahlberg L, et al. Cartilage matrix metabolism in osteoarthritis: markers in synovial fluid, serum, and urine. Clin Biochem 1992; 25: 167–74

148. Thompson PW, Spector TD, James IT, et al. Urinary collagen crosslinks reflect the radiographic severity of knee osteoarthritis. Br J Rheumatol 1992; 31: 759–61

149. Shinmei M, Ito K, Matsuyama S, et al. Joint fluid carboxy-terminal type II procollagen peptide as a marker of cartilage collagen biosynthesis. Osteoarthritis Cartilage 1993; 1: 121–8

150. MacDonald AG, McHenry P, Robins SP, Reid DM. Relationship of urinary pyridinium crosslinks to disease extent and activity in osteoarthritis. Br J Rheumatol 1994; 33: 16–19

151. Otterness IG, Swindell AC, Zimmerer RO, et al. An analysis of 14 molecular markers for monitoring osteoarthritis: segregation of the markers into clusters and distinguishing osteoarthritis at baseline. Osteoarthritis Cartilage 2000; 8: 180–5

152. Otterness IG, Weiner E, Swindell AC, et al. An analysis of 14 molecular markers for monitoring osteoarthritis. Relationship of the markers to clinical end-points. Osteoarthritis Cartilage 2001; 9: 224–31

153. DeGroot J, Bank RA, Tchetverikov I, et al. Molecular markers for osteoarthritis: the road ahead. Curr Opin Rheumatol 2002; 14: 585–9

4

Pathophysiology of osteoarthritis

Anthony J Freemont

PATHOLOGICAL DEFINITION OF OSTEOARTHRITIS

It is now recognized that osteoarthritis (OA) is a common name given to a group of disorders of synovial (diarthrodial) joints with a similar macroscopic morphology. The characteristic morphology (loss of articular cartilage, subchondral bone sclerosis, osteophyte formation and synovial hypertrophy) probably represents the final common outcome of a variety of pathogenic mechanisms that lead, ultimately, to joint failure.

To understand fully the pathogenesis and pathophysiology of OA requires an understanding of the anatomy and biology of the synovial joint.

THE NORMAL ANATOMY OF SYNOVIAL JOINTS

Structure and stability

Synovial joints allow very complex movements by virtue of their structure. The bone ends are not in contact but are covered by hyaline cartilage (Figure 4.1). Motion between the two cartilages is facilitated by the lubricating action of synovial fluid, a remarkable body fluid that is effectively a liquid tissue in which the matrix consists of a transudate of plasma supplemented by hyaluronans.[1] Unlike fibrous and cartilaginous joints, in which the stability of the joint comes from the bones being directly attached by the material forming the joint, diarthrodial joints gain their stability from a complex of structures surrounding the joint, including the capsule, ligaments and muscles. These structures prevent separation of the two bone ends. To give stability, a suitable 'spacer' is required

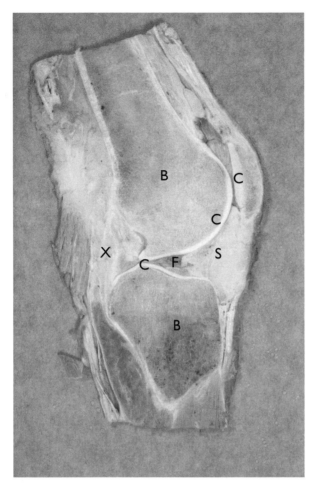

Figure 4.1 A section through a human knee, showing the bone (B), cartilage (C), synovium space (S) containing synovial fluid (F) and capsule (X)

to bring the capsule and ligaments under tension. Cartilage acts as the spacer. This is made possible by its natural tendency to expand, a function of the swelling pressure generated by one of its molecular components, proteoglycan (see below). Thus, the two opposing forces of the cartilage trying to push the bone apart, and the capsule, ligaments and muscle preventing it, maintains stability. It follows that should the cartilage reduce in amount or the capsule and ligaments become lax, the joint will become unstable. Instability *per se* may lead to an increased risk of developing OA or be a consequence of it.

Synovium and synovial fluid

The space created by the capsule is lined in part by the cartilage over the bone ends, and elsewhere by synovium. Synovium is a specialized lining tissue found in a number of sites where there is an interface between solid and liquid connective tissue matrices. It consists of an incomplete surface cell layer of synoviocytes made up of two cell populations: fibroblast-derived cells specialized to produce hyaluronans; and macrophages that phagocytose debris shed from the cartilage and synovium into the synovial fluid. The synovial subintima (the layer of tissue immediately below the synoviocyte layer) contains the only blood vessels and nerves within the lining tissues of the joint.

Articular cartilage

Articular cartilage covers the bone ends of synovial joints. The cartilage is made up of two distinct layers (Figure 4.2): a relatively thick outer layer consisting of

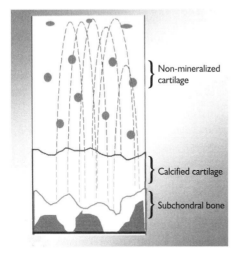
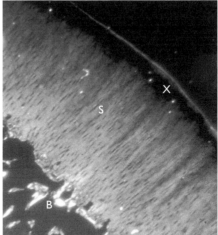

Figure 4.2 A composite consisting of a diagram of a cross-section of cartilage, to show its major components, and a micrograph taken using a polarizing microscope. In the diagram, note the relationship and relative thickness of the mineralized and non-mineralized cartilage, the morphology of the chondrocytes and the loops of type II collagen fibres. In the photomicrograph, the silken sheen of the ordered type II collagen fibres (S) overlies the bone (B), which can be recognized by its lamellar structure. The surface region of the cartilage (X) lacks 'sheen' because of the orientation of the collagen fibres

91

non-mineralized cartilage; and a relatively thin inner layer consisting of calcified cartilage at the interface between the cartilage and the cortex-like bone plate on which the cartilage sits, and to which it is attached by collagen fibres. The non-mineralized cartilage itself has two zones. There is a thin outer zone, in which the cells are flattened and the collagen fibres (see below) are running parallel to the surface, and the main body of the cartilage in which the chondrocytes are rounded, the collagen fibres run at right angles to the surface and the matrix is rich in proteoglycans.

Chondrocytes usually lead a solitary existence within spaces in the matrix called lacunae. They obtain nutrients and chemical messages by molecular diffusion and load-induced bulk transport through the extracellular matrix (ECM). The lacunae have a complex lining comprising a number of specialized molecules, including type VI collagen,[2] that effectively surrounds them with a protective 'shell'. In very general terms, chondrocytes have the ability to produce and remodel the ECM of cartilage. The biosynthetic activity of the chondrocytes varies with their position within the cartilage, the most active cells lying within the mid-zone.[3] The ECM has a hierarchy of structures, from the apparently homogeneous material seen macroscopically to the ordered molecular mixture at the submicroscopic level.[4]

At the molecular level, cartilage has two major components: type II collagen and proteoglycans. The pioneering work of Scott has defined how these elements relate to one another, and their role in maintaining the function and shape of cartilage.[5–7]

Type II collagen is a fibrillar collagen. The fibrils are arranged in such a way as to form loops, the free ends of which are attached to the bone, and the tops of the loops form the surface layers of the cartilage. These loops of type II collagen fibres effectively bind the cartilage down to the bone. The proteoglycans (of which the most abundant is aggrecan) are highly hydrophilic and swell by imbibation of water. The loops of type II collagen limit the swelling of the highly hydrophilic proteoglycans and, when both components are present in optimal amounts, the two opposing forces make the cartilage resilient.

PATHOLOGY OF OSTEOARTHRITIS

Symptoms and radiological changes

The joint derangement in OA, with subsequent diminished movement and chronic pain, is progressive, but the course of the disorder is often punctuated by episodes of acute pain and swelling.[8] Sequential radiological features of the disease include gradual loss of joint space (narrowing of the gap between the bones on the two sides of the joint, as a result of cartilage loss); formation of cysts beneath the articulating surfaces; progressive subarticular bone sclerosis (an increase in the amount of bone at the bone ends adjacent to the affected joint); and formation of bony buttresses (osteophytes) at the periphery of the joint.[9]

The pathology and pathophysiology of OA must be considered within the context of the clinical and radiological features of the disease, mainly because the pathology is, of necessity, a series of snapshots of a dynamic process. When piecing together the progress of the pathological changes, it is therefore essential that the single time point of the pathological image is interpreted with the dynamic radiological and clinical features. Animal models, studied in controlled cohorts, are the one way to follow the progression of the pathology of OA but, as in all animal models, there is always concern that the animal and Man are not identical, and that disease processes and tissue changes may not be directly transferable between species.[10] The following is a description of the pathological progression, based on a combination of studies of human tissue and relevant animal models.

Articular cartilage

The initial changes in the cartilage are focal (Figure 4.3). The first change noticed histologically is a loss of proteoglycan from the superficial layers of the cartilage (Figure 4.4). This stage is thought to be reversible. The reduction in proteoglycan disturbs the balance between the swelling pressure of the proteoglycan and the tension of the type II collagen fibres. It is thought that this 'softens' the cartilage, which is then less able to withstand loading, resulting in traumatic damage to the type II collagen framework. It is believed that damage to the type II collagen fibres cannot be spontaneously repaired. Damage to the collagen fibres leads to the development of superficial splits (fissures) that propagate both parallel with and at right angles to the surface (Figure 4.5).

Gradual cartilage damage and loss occur focally, propagating downwards towards the bone and laterally away from the initial area of damage. Ultimately, this results in an area of the articular surface from which cartilage is lost completely and bone/calcified cartilage exposed (Figure 4.6). This area is surrounded by a region of damaged cartilage.

These changes are usually present over both opposing articular surfaces, and the joint becomes an articulation between two pieces of bone. The exposed bone

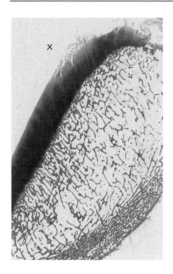

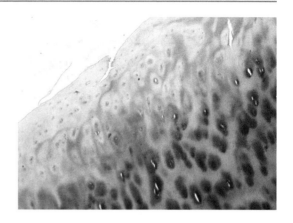

Figure 4.4 Photomicrograph of the earliest cartilage changes of OA. There is loss of proteoglycans (the tissue stains blue/purple where proteoglycans are present), and a small fissure has developed in the surface of the cartilage (H&E 200×)

Figure 4.3 Whole-mount section of patella, showing how the earliest cartilage changes of OA (marked X) are focal and superficial

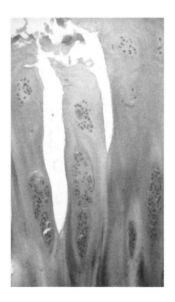

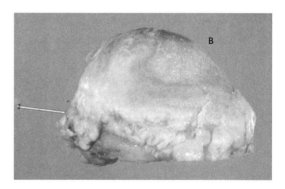

Figure 4.6 A macro-photograph of a femoral head with advanced osteoarthritic change. Eburnated bone (B) is seen centrally, surrounded by abnormal cartilage. The pin marks the site of osteophytes

Figure 4.5 Fissures extending into the cartilage at right angles to the surface. Note the chondrocyte clones (H&E 200×)

is worn down to form a smooth hard surface, a process known as eburnation. Between them the eburnated bone and the damaged cartilage produce an abnormal shape to the articular surface and, because cartilage has been lost, the joint becomes unstable. The eburnated bone is often pocked by small areas of fibrous tissue and fibrocartilage.

Chondrocytes

It is possible to recognize four different types of chondrocyte in osteoarthritic cartilage: (1) normal chondrocytes manufacturing type II collagen and aggrecan; (2) chondrocytes singly and in clusters, or clones, which have undergone partial de-differentiation to a fibroblast-like phenotype synthesizing type I and type III collagen; (3) hypertrophic chondrocytes, which have adopted a phenotype similar to that seen in the foetal cartilage and growth plates, and which synthesize type X collagen, a non-fibrillar collagen associated with the process of endochondral ossification (formation of bone from cartilage); and (4) apoptotic chondrocytes – chondrocytes dying using energy-dependent mechanisms.

Repair

Although it does not seem possible for cartilage to be restored to its original state by its indigenous chondrocytes once the collagen network has been damaged, repair of sorts is attempted. At the periphery of the joint a repair process can be seen as a cellular layer of cartilage extending over, and sometimes dissecting into, the existing damaged cartilage. This extrinsically repaired cartilage is usually much more cellular than the pre-existing articular cartilage, and the chondrocytes are unevenly distributed through the matrix. On polarizing microscopy, which enables the molecular orientation of collagen molecules to be visualized, discontinuity between the collagen network of the repaired cartilage and that of the pre-existing cartilage can be easily seen. As an aside, this demonstrates the main problem of naturally and artificially repairing articular cartilage, namely the difficulty of biointegrating new tissue with the old residual cartilage. Biointegration is essential if the cartilage is to successfully withstand prolonged loading.

That the residual chondrocytes are attempting to rebuild the matrix can be shown by the increased uptake of radioactive sulphate (a marker of sulphated proteoglycan synthesis) sometimes seen in OA cartilage. This is most pronounced adjacent to fissures. Despite this, the amount of proteoglycan in the matrix of OA cartilage is decreased. This apparent paradox is explained by increased leaching of the newly synthesized proteoglycan into the synovial fluid because of decreased binding of the newly synthesized proteoglycans to the defective collagen fibrils.

The presence of small islands of fibrocartilage within the eburnated bone has already been described. These result from damage to the bone, often with exposure of the marrow. The marrow contains mesenchymal stem cells, multipotent cells with the ability to differentiate into any connective tissue. In the environment of the OA joint they develop into small nodules of fibrocartilage. Dependent upon the load environment, the fibrocartilage can (but rarely does) grow over the eburnated surface and may form a complete covering of fibrocartilagenous repair tissue.

Other structures within the joint

The changes within the osteoarthritic joint are not restricted to the articular cartilage. The disease process also affects the subchondral and marginal bone, the synovium and the synovial fluid.

Subchondral bone

There is a continuing debate as to whether the earliest changes of OA take place within the subchondral bone. There is evidence[11] that the first changes detectable in OA are thickening and an increased density of the subchondral bone plate, raising the suggestion that this might be the initiating event, leading to the characteristic cartilage changes of OA by interfering with the flow of nutrients into the articular cartilage from the adjacent bone marrow. There is no doubt that in most cases of OA there is a generalized anabolic effect in bone. The normal balance between osteoblastic and osteoclastic activity (coupling) that maintains a constant bone mass is lost and, as a consequence, there is a marked increase in bone cell activity generally, but with an excess of osteoblastic bone deposition, leading to subchondral bone sclerosis and osteophyte formation (Figure 4.7).

Osteophytes

It is believed that instability causes osteophyte formation, but the exact mechanism(s) is/are still unknown. The net effect of osteophyte formation is to

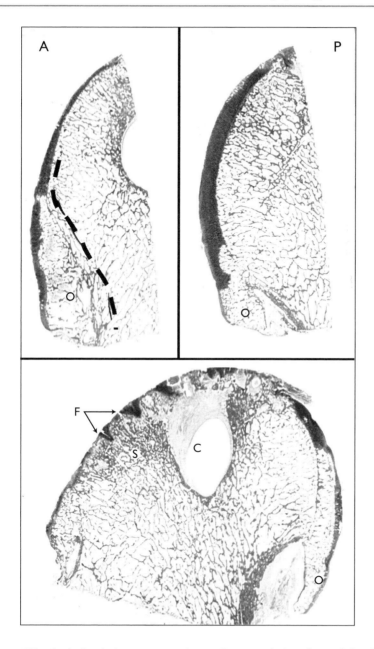

Figure 4.7 Histological whole-mount sections of osteoarthritic femoral head. The larger section is in the medio-lateral plane and the other two represent anterior (A) and posterior (P) slices. There is marked subchondral bone sclerosis (S), a large cyst (C), fibrocartilagenous plugs in the subchondral bone (F) and osteophytes (O). The previous line of the femoral head is marked with a dashed line and delineated by a thin line of residual purple cartilage. The osteophyte is covered by cartilage

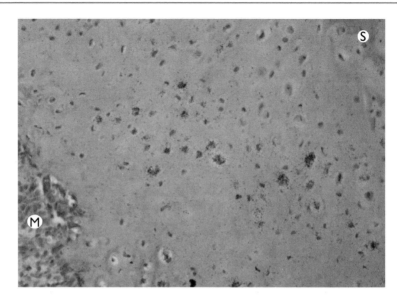

Figure 4.8 A section of femoral head cartilage at the root of an osteophyte, showing a black *in situ* hybridization reaction product for type X collagen gene in the mid-zone of the cartilage. The surface (S) of the cartilage is to the right and above, and marrow (M) can be seen at the bottom left of the image (150x)

increase stability by increasing the size of the articulating surface. There is a growing body of evidence that points towards the formation of some osteophytes being due to regression of the phenotype of mid-zone chondrocytes near the edge of the cartilage towards that seen normally in foetal development. The mid-zone chondrocytes become hypertrophic, express the type X collagen gene[12] (Figure 4.8) and initiate: (1) calcification within the mid-zone of the cartilage; (2) ingrowth of capillaries; and (3) endochondral ossification. As the disease progresses, this zone of new bone formation extends centrally. Once initiated, progressive new bone formation within the cartilage separates the cartilage into two layers, one of which comes to lie on the surface of the osteophyte and the other appears to be buried deep within the bone, in the line of the original articular surface. These are separated by the bone of the osteophyte (Figure 4.7).

Other osteophytes form by endochondral ossification from foci of chondroid metaplasia at the enthesis (the junction of capsular and ligamentous insertions into bone) at the joint margins. They are almost certainly the result of traction injuries secondary to joint instability. In this type of osteophyte, the cartilage overlying the bone overgrowth is usually hypercellular, and has a similar appearance to a growth plate.

Bone necrosis

Normally the subchondral bone is protected from load by the overlying cartilage. Eburnated bone is not protected in this way and is prone to local pressure necrosis. This affects both the bone and the underlying marrow, so that the marrow cannot repair by stimulation of marrow stem cells. These areas of necrosis are usually very small.

Bone cysts

Bone cysts or geodes are a feature of advanced OA (Figure 4.7). They form as a consequence of synovial fluid entering the bone marrow. Unlike cartilage, bone is naturally permeated by narrow channels, either in the form of Haversian systems or the canaliculi linking osteocyte lacunae. These channels make convenient routes for synovial fluid to be forced under pressure from the joint cavity into the marrow. Once in the marrow, the synovial fluid elicits a bipolar reaction with osteoclastic bone destruction and osteoblastic bone deposition. Ultimately, this leads to the formation of a cyst within the bone, containing fibrous or myxoid tissue, and lined by sclerotic bone and fibrous tissue.

Synovium

In OA, the synovium is thrown into finger-like folds or villi. There is an increase in the number and size of synoviocytes in the synovial membrane (Figure 4.9). In many cases, particularly early in the course of the disease, the synovium appears inflamed, due to increased blood flow through the synovium and perivascular oedema associated with a mast cell infiltrate.[13] As disease advances, there is progressive synovial fibrosis. Whilst there is never the florid accumulation of lymphocytes and plasma cells in the villi and synovial subintima that is seen in the inflammatory arthropathies, not infrequently, particularly in advanced OA, perivascular aggregates of lymphocytes are seen and, more rarely, occasional plasma cells (see last section – 'Immune system activation and the pathogenesis of OA'). Occasionally, bone and cartilage debris enters the synovium and elicits a macrophage response. Aggregates of calcium pyrophosphate crystals are also sometimes seen in the synovium.

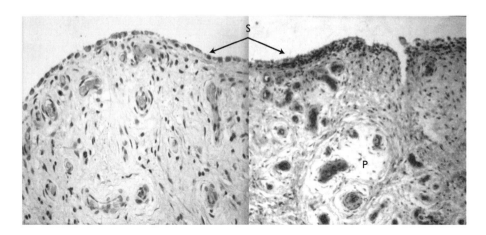

Figure 4.9 A composite showing normal synovium on the left and OA synovium on the right. Note the increased number of synoviocytes (S) in the OA case compared with the incomplete layer of flat cells in the normal case. The subintima of the OA cartilage is oedematous (note the perivascular clear zone (P) made by the collection of oedema fluid). (H&E – normal 250x, OA 150x)

Synovial fluid

In OA, the synovial fluid often increases in volume, particularly during the flares described above. This is due to increased 'leakiness' of synovial capillaries, possibly mediated by mast cell products. The fluid remains viscid but contains debris (e.g. articular cartilage, pyrophosphate and hydroxyapatite crystals, bone and fragments of synovial villi) shed into the fluid from the deteriorating articular surfaces and joint lining. The cell count is always low, never exceeding 1000 cells/mm^3.[1]

THE MOLECULAR BIOLOGY OF NORMAL AND OSTEOARTHRITIC CARTILAGE

The progressive unravelling of the pathophysiology of OA is one of the most remarkable stories in modern biology. It completely turned around thinking about connective tissue metabolism, 'degeneration' and the biology of inflammation. It has focused on articular cartilage and the interactions between chondrocytes and their matrix, but now involves the altered biology of the synovium, and is beginning to explain the changes seen in bone. In very general terms, in OA, the chondrocytes switch from an anabolic to a catabolic phenotype, in a series of processes driven by locally synthesized cytokines.

Turnover of the extracellular matrix of cartilage

Chondrocytes are responsible for making and maintaining the ECM of cartilage. The ECM, in turn, conveys information about the local environment to the chondrocytes. The chondrocyte is attached to the inner surface of its lacunae by cell adhesion molecules called integrins[14] and, through these adhesions, it can 'sense' load and the chemical composition of its matrix. To understand fully the interactions of chondrocytes and the ECM in OA it is necessary to first appreciate the homeostatic mechanisms operating in normal cartilage.

Despite superficial appearances, cartilage matrix is continually being renewed. Tritiated proline and radiosulphate uptake studies show just how much collagen and sulphated proteoglycan, respectively, are being synthesized by chondrocytes, particularly within the deeper two-thirds of the cartilage.[3] To make way for newly synthesized matrix, old ECM has to be removed; this is achieved by enzymic digestion. Matrix-degrading enzymes are synthesized as latent proenzymes, and then activated where required, also by enzymic digestion. It is believed that two families of degrading enzymes are particularly involved in cartilage turnover: the matrix metalloproteinases (MMPs) and the ADAMTs, a subgroup of MMPs set apart by having disintegrin as well as metalloproteinase activity, and which also contain the thrombospondin motif. Key members of these two families are MMP13 (a specific type II collagenase)[15] and ADAMTs 1, 4 and 5 (which are specific aggrecanases).[16]

As indicated, the activity of these enzymes is highly regulated. In keeping with other molecules, their production is regulated by DNA transcription and RNA translation into proenzymes. The active enzymes have to be produced from the proenzyme, necessitating the presence of an activating enzyme. There are a number of candidates, including specific membrane-bound MMPs, known as MT-MMPs, and families of serine- and cysteine-dependent proteinases, such as plasminogen activator and cathepsin B.[17]

There are also specific inhibitors of these MMPs and ADAMTs, most notably the TIMPs (tissue inactivator of metalloproteinases). Three (TIMP-1, TIMP-2 and TIMP-3) are believed to be central to the regulation of cartilage degradation.[17]

The regulation of cartilage matrix synthesis and degradation is such a complex system that it is hardly surprising to find that studies of OA have implicated derangement of several different components in the initiation and propagation of cartilage damage in OA. It is perceived that the major problem is a combination of a failure to manufacture the normal amount and type of matrix, together with increased breakdown of matrix by aggrecanases and type II collagenases.[18] Chondrocytes in OA synthesize non-cartilage collagens (notably types I and III) and abnormal proteoglycans. There is also increased enzymic breakdown of cartilage due to: deficiencies of TIMPs;[19] the presence of novel TIMPs;[20] up-regulation of cathepsin B;[21] and aberrant production of MMP-13. From such observations have arisen possibilities for managing OA by interfering with these abnormal metabolic pathways.

Growth factors, cytokines and other soluble mediators in cartilage remodelling and OA

Whilst it is entirely reasonable to note that turnover of matrix in normal and diseased cartilage is a function of expression of genes responsible for the synthesis and breakdown of ECM molecules, it would be unthinking to assume that these molecules are spontaneous products of chondrocytes. Increasingly, interest has turned to the role of molecular regulators, such as cytokines and growth factors, in the regulation of chondrocyte function.

Growth factors and hormones

Cartilage ECM synthesis and repair are regulated through insulin-like growth factors 1 and 2 (IGF-1 and -2)[22] and their regulators, IGF binding proteins (IGFBPs).[23] Response of differentiated chondrocytes to IGFs is promoted by growth hormone (GH). OA chondrocytes seem less responsive to IGFs, and there are also aberrations of serum GH and IGF and chondrocyte synthesis of IGFBP in OA patients, perhaps implicating disturbances of the GH/IGF/IGFBP axis in the cartilage damage in OA.[24] It is also worth noting that the GH/IGF axis is key to the development and function of osteoblasts, which may explain both cartilage breakdown and bone production in the pathology of OA.

Cytokines

Cytokines have taken on an important perspective as process mediators in cartilage injury and repair.[25] Both isoforms of the cytokine interleukin-1 (IL-1)

– IL-1α and IL-1β – play key roles in altering the turnover of articular cartilage ECM. Both will up-regulate production of MMPs, and IL-1β will suppress TIMP synthesis. In the osteoarthritic joint there is increased production of IL-1, and the synoviocyte layer has been identified as the site of its synthesis. That a so-called 'pro-inflammatory cytokine' can be produced outside of classical inflammatory processes is part of a realization that cytokines are not only pro-inflammatory but have a fundamental regulatory role in homeostasis. The discovery of the significance of IL-1 in OA has also given rise to the proposal that IL-1 antagonists, such as IL-1 receptor antagonist or the soluble IL-1 receptor, might be used to inhibit progression of cartilage damage in OA joints.[26]

Other cytokines, including tumour necrosis factor-α (TNF-α), IL-6, IL-8, IL-4, IL-10, IL-13 and interferon-γ, have been implicated in the regulation of cartilage metabolism in health and disease, but rather like the proposed central role for TNF in rheumatoid disease, IL-1 has been suggested by some as a 'master regulator' of the joint changes in OA.[27]

No cytokine can function without the expression of its receptor(s) by the target cell. In OA, articular chondrocytes express the activating IL-1 type 1 receptor on their cell membranes. They also express the p55 and p75 receptors for TNF-α, and there has been recent interest in this cytokine as a possible mediator and therapeutic target in OA. Interestingly, IGF-1 and transforming growth factor-β1 (TGF-β1; a cytokine known to have a role in embryonic cartilage development and in wound healing) inhibit TNF-α-mediated MMP production.

Other soluble mediators

Nitric oxide (NO) has been found in increased amounts in OA synovial fluid and synovium, and in the serum of patients with OA.[28] There are remarkable links between it and other factors implicated in OA. For instance, IL-1β augments production of NO by articular chondrocytes; and NO can activate articular cartilage MMPs.[29] There are inhibitors of NO production already in therapeutic use in other disorders, and their application in human OA appears only a matter of time.

Summary

Combining all these and many more data has given rise to the concept that a chemokine network centred on IL-1 and TNF, and mediated by other pro-inflammatory cytokines and soluble mediators such as NO, lies at the heart of the processes that lead to cartilage damage and other joint changes that characterize OA, and could be a potent target for novel therapies.[30,31]

Chondrocyte apoptosis

One of the major features of OA is the death of articular chondrocytes by apoptosis.[32] There is an anomaly here in that, overall, the number of chondrocytes within OA cartilage may not be reduced because those chondrocytes that do not die reproduce to form large lacunae containing many chondrocytes; however, the number of lacunae containing viable cells decreases dramatically in cartilage affected by the processes of OA. Clearly, loss of the elements that form matrix will have a significant impact on its synthesis but, on the other hand, will also limit the production of degrading enzymes. The one difference is that whilst proenzymes can diffuse through the matrix away from viable cells, it is not thought that matrix molecules have the same mobility.

Apoptosis can be induced by IL-1, TNF and NO amongst others.[33] It is mediated through two pathways: one (the extrinsic pathway) based on the cell membrane and activated by TNF, and the other (intrinsic pathway) by cytochrome c released from mitochondria. Apoptosis is inhibited by a group of intracellular molecules called Bcl-2. Bcl-2 production is lower in OA cartilage than in normal cartilage. Intriguingly, Bcl-2 is linked with the production of aggrecan, making the relationship between cytokines and chondrocyte function even more complicated than it first appeared.[34]

As intimated above, biological anti-cytokines are proposed therapeutic agents for the management of cartilage damage in OA. If chondrocyte loss through apoptosis has as significant a role in the cartilage damage of OA as some believe, then the intracellular pathways of apoptosis might also be important targets in the management of OA. The processes of apoptosis working through protein kinases focus on the transcription factor NF-κB.[35] There are contradictory data on the role of NF-κB in apoptosis. Rapid induction appears to be pro-apoptotic, whereas steady production appears to be anti-apoptotic. In this context, it is interesting to note that naturally occurring molecules such as hyaluronic acid, chondroitin sulphate and glucosamine augment NF-κB activity, perhaps offering a biological explanation for the suggested efficacy of these molecules in OA.

LOAD, CHONDROCYTE FUNCTION AND OSTEOARTHRITIS

During normal movement, articular cartilage is exposed to very high compressive loads. Cartilage is uniquely designed to resist load, and the chondrocytes are protected from load by the structure of the lacunae. Nevertheless, the lacunae are deformable in a manner that is dependent upon the load. Through the integrin cell adhesion molecules, chondrocytes respond to load signals. Through the exacting work of Salter and his colleagues[36] we have an idea of the molecular mechanisms by which chondrocytes recognize and respond to load. His group has shown that human articular chondrocytes use the $\alpha_5\beta_1$ integrin as a mechanoreceptor. Mechanical stimulation of this receptor activates a signal cascade involving stretch-activated ion channels, the actin microfibrils of the cytoskeleton and tyrosine phosphorylation of focal adhesion complex molecules. This, in turn, leads to synthesis of IL-4, which acts in an autocrine manner inducing synthesis of aggrecan and decreasing production of MMP RNAs. This is one explanation for the high content of proteoglycan in areas of cartilage exposed to high load. These and other studies[37] have demonstrated, in cartilage explants from normal joints, that cyclical loading stimulates matrix synthesis, whereas static loading inhibits it. It is also well established *in vitro* that normal chondrocyte function is dependent on intermittent loading, without which matrix synthesis stops, suggesting that cartilage homeostasis is dependent upon normal joint usage, including repetitive low-impact loading.[38]

There is a body of evidence indicating that abnormal loading of the joint will precipitate the cycle of events that leads to OA. Thus, repetitive high-impact loading, obesity and occupations involving demanding physical activity are risk factors for the development of OA. Abnormally directed load, as much as abnormal quantities of load, may also lead to OA. Examples include abnormal gait, whether related to skeletal development such as skeletal dysplasias, or lifestyle, such as the wearing of high-heeled shoes. Abnormal response of cartilage to load may also explain: the increased propensity to develop OA in disorders such as ochronosis, where the physical properties of cartilage affect its ability to resist loading; and the link between subchondral bone sclerosis and osteoarthritic changes in the overlying cartilage, on the basis of altered resilience of the cartilage/bone-plate complex.

The molecular mechanisms linking the pathophysiology of OA to abnormal loading are not yet established, but it is now recognized that abnormal loading will induce IL-1 and MMP production[39] in joints, and there is some evidence that abnormalities in chondroprotective mechanotransduction pathways may contribute to disease progression.

CHONDROCYTE SENESCENCE AND OSTEOARTHRITIS

The incidence of OA directly correlates with age. This is hardly surprising as OA is a disorder that, once acquired, is irreversible and progressive. However, this association has led investigators to examine chondrocytes in aging cartilage and in OA for evidence of senescence. Both with increasing age and in OA the ability of chondrocytes to maintain cartilage matrix integrity is impaired. Recent work suggests that progressive chondrocyte senescence, marked by expression of the senescence-associated enzyme β-galactosidase, reduction of telomere length and mitochondrial degeneration due to oxidative damage, causes this loss of chondrocyte function. Senescence also increases the risk of a cell entering apoptosis. The discovery of an association between OA and the development of senescent phenotype by articular chondrocytes raises the possibility that novel approaches to the management of OA might include strategies that slow or even reverse the progression of chondrocyte senescence.[40,41]

GENETICS AND OSTEOARTHRITIS

Evidence suggests that genetic factors play a major role in OA. The familial occurrence of Heberden's nodes, a characteristic feature of primary generalized OA (the most common form of inherited OA), was described as long ago as 1941.[42] It has been estimated that the genetic influence is probably in excess of 50% for certain types of OA, and first-degree relatives have two or three times the risk of developing OA.[43] Simple Mendelian inheritance has been identified for a single gene mutation in some very rare familial forms of OA, but the genetic basis of the common forms of OA is polygenic and still poorly characterized.

The precise nature of the gene changes in OA is still being investigated, and many sequences have been suggested as being potential important candidates for OA-inducing mutations. Some relate to risk factors, such as obesity, and others come directly from an improved understanding of the molecular biology of OA. These involve either genes encoding structural components of the ECM of cartilage, such as type II collagen, or molecules such as TGF-β, which are key members of the metabolic pathways of articular chondrocytes or the cells of subchondral bone.

There is conclusive evidence that mutations in the alpha 1 chain of type II collagen are present in members of some families with primary generalized OA, whereas there is equally conclusive evidence that in other families there is no such mutation. Other ECM molecules have been considered, including other types of collagen, notably collagens IX, X and XI, aggrecan and decorin. Amongst candidate genes associated more with bone and cartilage cell function[44] are those encoding the vitamin D receptor, TGF-β, the estrogen receptor, TNF and IL-1.

IMMUNE SYSTEM ACTIVATION AND THE PATHOGENESIS OF OSTEOARTHRITIS

There has been a concerted, if spasmodic, interest in the role of immune-mediated events in the genesis of OA. These go beyond the now fully accepted cytokine-mediated events that have a central role in the disorder. Immune-mediated events have been implicated in both the initiation and progression of OA, and could well become therapeutic targets.[45] Antigens capable of stimulating both the humoral and cell-mediated arms of the immune system have been identified in cartilage; they include the central and link protein groups of proteoglycans, particularly those associated with chondroitin sulphate attachment areas. The synovial fluid of patients with OA has been shown to contain such antigens.

It is believed that chondrocytes occupy an immune privileged site within their lacunae deep within cartilage. Cartilage damage may expose the cell membranes of the chondrocytes in OA to the immune system, which may explain why some patients with OA demonstrate cellular and humoral immune reactions to epitopes in chondrocyte membranes.

Immunohistochemistry of cartilage is plagued by the fact that chondrocytes also exhibit antigen-presenting properties. In OA, articular chondrocytes have been shown to express the human leukocyte antigens DP, DQ and DR; they also have increased expression of CD80 and CD86, which are required for activation of T lymphocytes. On the basis of this and other studies, it has been suggested that in OA the chondrocytes of damaged cartilage can act as antigen-presenting cells for T lymphocytes and initiate a cell-mediated immune response. This may explain the presence of T lymphocytes within the synovium in end-stage OA. Both CD4 and CD8 cells are present in the subintima, and Th1 cells outnumber Th2 cells five to one. The lymphocytic aggregates show markers of early, intermediate and late T-cell activation, as well as the Th1 cytokines IL-2 and interferon-γ.

Patients with OA have also been shown to have antibodies against chondrocyte membrane proteins, cartilage proteins and proteoglycan link protein in their serum and synovial fluids, suggesting a potential role for humoral immunity in the pathogenesis of OA.[46] It has long been held that such antibodies might be deposited on the surface of the fissures in osteoarthritic cartilage and initiate cytotoxic events;[47] this may be through fixing complement, and certainly complement deposits are found within the tissues of osteoarthritic joints. This may be an important observation, as activated C1 has the ability to break down collagen. Potentially more intriguing, but still not fully understood, is the ability of chondrocytes[48] themselves to synthesize components of complement.

References

1. Freemont AJ, Denton J. Atlas of Synovial Fluid Cytopathology. Dordrecht: Kluwer Academic Publishers, 1991

2. Soder S, Hambach L, Lissner R, et al. Ultrastructural localization of type VI collagen in normal adult and osteoarthritic human articular cartilage. Osteoarthritis Cartilage 2002; 10: 464–70

3. Marles PJ, Hoyland JA, Parkinson R, Freemont AJ. Demonstration of variation in chondrocyte activity in different zones of articular cartilage – an assessment of the value of in-situ hybridisation. Int J Exp Pathol 1991; 72: 171–82

4. Foster JE, Maciewicz RA, Tabener A, et al. Structural periodicity in human articular cartilage: comparison between magnetic resonance imaging and histological findings. Osteoarthritis Cartilage 1999; 7: 480–5

5. Scott JE. Elasticity in extracellular matrix shape modules of tendon, cartilage etc. A sliding proteoglycan-filament model. J Physiol 2003; 553: 335–43

6. Scott JE. Structure and function in extracellular matrices depend on interactions between anionic glycosaminoglycans. Pathol Biol (Paris) 2001; 49: 284–9

7. Scott JE, Dyne KM, Thomlinson AM, et al. Human cells unable to express decoron produced disorganized extracellular matrix lacking "shape modules" (interfibrillar proteoglycan bridges). Exp Cell Res 1998; 243: 59–66

8. Kellgren JH. Osteoarthrosis in patients and populations. Br Med J 1961; 2: 1–6

9. Lawrence J, Bremner BM, Bier F. Osteoarthrosis. Ann Rheum Dis 1966; 25: 1–2

10. Das-Gupta EP, Lyons TJ, Hoyland JA, et al. New histological observations in spontaneously developing osteoarthritis in the STR/ORT mouse, questioning its acceptability as a model of human osteoarthritis. Int J Exp Pathol 1993; 74: 627–34

11. Hunter DJ, Spector TD. The role of bone metabolism in osteoarthritis. Curr Rheumatol Rep 2003; 5: 15–19

12. Hoyland JA, Thomas JT, Donn R, et al. Distribution of type X collagen in normal and OA human cartilage. Bone Miner 1991; 15: 151–64

13. Dean G, Hoyland JA, Denton J, et al. Mast cells in the synovium and synovial fluid in osteoarthritis. Br J Rheumatol 1993; 32: 671–5

14. Ostergaard K, Salter DM, Petersen J, et al. Expression of alpha and beta subunits of the integrin superfamily in articular cartilage from macroscopically normal and osteoarthritic human femoral heads. Ann Rheum Dis 1998; 57: 303–8

15. Poole AR, Kobayashi M, Yasuda T, et al. Type II collagen degradation and its regulation in articular cartilage in osteoarthritis. Ann Rheum Dis 2002; 61 (Suppl 2): 78–81

16. Nagase H, Kashiwagi M. Aggrecanases and cartilage matrix degradation. Arthritis Res Ther 2003; 5: 94–103 [Epub 2003 Feb 14]

17. Smith RL. Degradative enzymes in osteoarthritis. Front Biosci 1999; 4: D704–12

18. Freemont AJ, Byers RJ, Taiwo YO, Hoyland JA. In situ zymographic localisation of type II collagen degrading activity in osteoarthritic human articular cartilage. Ann Rheum Dis 1999; 58: 357–65

19. Su S, Grover J, Roughley PJ, et al. Expression of the tissue inhibitor of metallo-proteinases (TIMP) gene family in normal and osteoarthritic joints. Rheumatol Int 1999; 18: 183–91

20. Huang W, Li WQ, Dehnade F, Zafarullah M. Tissue inhibitor of metallopro-teinases-4 (TIMP-4) gene expression is increased in human osteoarthritic femoral head cartilage. J Cell Biochem 2002; 85: 295–303

21. Buttle DJ, Handley CJ, Ilic MZ, et al. Inhibition of cartilage proteoglycan release by a specific inactivator of cathepsin B and an inhibitor of matrix metallopro-teinases. Evidence for two converging pathways of chondrocyte-mediated proteo-glycan degradation. Arthritis Rheum 1993; 36: 1709–17

22. Messai H, Duchossoy Y, Khatib AM, et al. Articular chondrocytes from aging rats respond poorly to insulin-like growth factor-1: an altered signaling pathway. Mech Ageing Dev 2000; 115: 21–37

23. Martin JA, Ellerbroek SM, Buckwalter JA. Age-related decline in chondrocyte response to insulin-like growth factor-I: the role of growth factor binding proteins. J Orthop Res 1997; 15: 491–8

24. Denko CW, Malemud CJ. Metabolic disturbances and synovial joint responses in osteoarthritis. Front Biosci 1999; 4: D686–93

25. Lotz M. Cytokines in cartilage injury and repair. Clin Orthop 2001; 391 (Suppl): S108–15

26. Goldring MB. Anticytokine therapy for osteoarthritis. Expert Opin Biol Ther 2001; 1: 817–29

27. Fernandes JC, Martel-Pelletier J, Pelletier JP. The role of cytokines in osteoarthritis pathophysiology. Biorheology 2002; 39: 237–46

28. Amin AR, Dave M, Attur M, Abramson SB. COX-2, NO, and cartilage damage and repair. Curr Rheumatol Rep 2000; 2: 447–53

29. Abramson SB, Attur M, Amin AR, Clancy R. Nitric oxide and inflammatory mediators in the perpetuation of osteoarthritis. Curr Rheumatol Rep 2001; 3: 535–41

30. Goldberg SH, Von Feldt JM, Lonner JH. Pharmacologic therapy for osteoarthritis. Am J Orthop 2002; 31: 673–80

31. Chikanza I, Fernandes L. Novel strategies for the treatment of osteoarthritis. Expert Opin Investig Drugs 2000; 9: 1499–1510

32. Goggs R, Carter SD, Schulze-Tanzil G, et al. Apoptosis and the loss of chondrocyte survival signals contribute to articular cartilage degradation in osteoarthritis. Vet J 2003; 166: 140–58

33. Lotz M, Hashimoto S, Kuhn K. Mechanisms of chondrocyte apoptosis. Osteoarthritis Cartilage 1999; 7: 389–91

34. Feng L, Balakir R, Precht P, Horton WE Jr. Bcl-2 regulates chondrocyte morphology and aggrecan gene expression independent of caspase activation and full apoptosis. J Cell Biochem 1999; 74: 576–86

35. Liacini A, Sylvester J, Li WQ, Zafarullah M. Inhibition of interleukin-1-stimulated MAP kinases, activating protein-1 (AP-1) and nuclear factor kappa B (NF-kappa B) transcription factors down-regulates matrix metalloproteinase gene expression in articular chondrocytes. Matrix Biol 2002; 21: 251–62

36. Millward-Sadler SJ, Wright MO, Lee H, et al. Integrin-regulated secretion of interleukin 4: a novel pathway of mechanotransduction in human articular chondrocytes. J Cell Biol 1999; 145: 183–9

37. Deschner J, Hofman CR, Piesco NP, Agarwal S. Signal transduction by mechanical strain in chondrocytes. Curr Opin Clin Nutr Metab Care 2003; 6: 289–93

38. Kerin A, Patwari P, Kuettner K, et al. Molecular basis of osteoarthritis: biomechanical aspects. Cell Mol Life Sci 2002; 59: 27–35

39. Honda K, Ohno S, Tanimoto K, et al. The effects of high magnitude cyclic tensile load on cartilage matrix metabolism in cultured chondrocytes. Eur J Cell Biol 2000; 79: 601–9

40. Martin JA, Buckwalter JA. Human chondrocyte senescence and osteoarthritis. Biorheology 2002; 39: 145–52

41. Price JS, Waters JG, Darrah C, et al. The role of chondrocyte senescence in osteoarthritis. Aging Cell 2002; 1: 57–65

42. Stecher RM. Heberden's nodes. Heredity in hypertrophic arthritis of the finger joints. Am J Med Sci 1941; 801–12

43. Spector TD, Cicuttini F, Baker J, Hart DJ. Genetic influences on osteoarthritis in women: a twin study. Br Med J 1996; 312: 940–4

44. Ghosh P, Smith M. Osteoarthritis, genetic and molecular mechanisms. Biogerontology 2002; 3: 85–8

45. Yuan GH, Masuko-Hongo K, Kato T, Nishioka K. Immunologic intervention in the pathogenesis of osteoarthritis. Arthritis Rheum 2003; 48: 602–11

46. Alsalameh S, Mollenhauer J, Hain N, et al. Cellular immune response toward human articular chondrocytes. T cell reactivities against chondrocyte and fibroblast membranes in destructive joint diseases. Arthritis Rheum 1990; 33: 1477–86

47. Jasin HE. Autoantibody specificities of immune complexes sequestered in articular cartilage of patients with rheumatoid arthritis and osteoarthritis. Arthritis Rheum 1985; 28: 241–8

48. Bradley K, North J, Saunders D, et al. Synthesis of classical pathway complement components by chondrocytes. Immunology 1996; 88: 648–56

5

Non-pharmacological management of osteoarthritis

Leena Sharma

INTRODUCTION

Osteoarthritis (OA) is clinically manifest in a substantial subset of the population; for example, it is estimated that 12% of Americans between the ages of 25 and 75 years have clinical signs and symptoms of OA.[1] The increase in the prevalence of symptomatic OA with age, coupled with the inadequacy of current symptom-relieving treatment and lack of disease-modifying treatment options, contributes to the overall burden of OA.

An array of non-pharmacological interventions for OA have been described (Table 5.1), each in various stages of development, investigation and application. Such interventions capitalize on knowledge of the causes of symptoms, disease progression and disability in patients with OA. Many non-pharmacological interventions are low-cost, incorporate self-management approaches and are home-based; as such, they may have a substantial public health impact.

Some non-pharmacological interventions for OA may ultimately be shown to contribute to secondary prevention (prevention of disease progression). At present, these approaches are applied predominantly to support tertiary prevention, i.e. to reduce symptoms and prevent disability. We recently reported on determinants of poor physical function over 3 years in people with knee OA using the WOMAC and chair stand performance.[2] Several factors identified are amenable to non-pharmacological intervention strategies: varus–valgus laxity (odds ratio (OR), adjusted for age, body mass index (BMI), knee pain intensity, disease severity, 1.58/3°); 0–18-month increase in knee pain intensity (adjusted OR/20 mm visual analogue scale (VAS) 1.48); SF36 mental health (adjusted OR 0.58/5 points); self-efficacy (adjusted OR 0.80/5 points); social support (adjusted

Table 5.1 Potential non-pharmacological therapies

Psychosocial
  Enhance self-efficacy
  Education
  Teach coping skills
  Improve social support
  Treat anxiety and depression
Physical activity, exercise and physical therapy to maintain
  Aerobic capacity and conditioning
  Strength
Occupational therapy
Treat local factors
  Inserts/insoles
  Footwear adjustment
  Bracing
  Other orthoses (e.g. neoprene sleeves)
  Enhance proprioceptive acuity
Weight loss if overweight
Acupuncture

OR 0.85/10 points); and aerobic exercise per week (adjusted OR 0.84/60 min).[2] We have also found that with an increase in the number of malaligned knees (i.e. from 0 to 1 to 2), there was a steady increase in the likelihood of poor physical function outcome.[3]

Recent studies and reviews of exercise, weight loss, education, inserts, footwear, bracing, therapeutic ultrasound, acupuncture and pulsed electromagnetic field therapy will be highlighted in this overview. For many of these interventions, further investigation is necessary to define precisely their place in OA management.

GUIDELINES FOR MANAGEMENT OF OSTEOARTHRITIS

Four sets of guidelines for the management of lower-limb OA (American College of Rheumatology (ACR),[4] European League Against Rheumatism,[5] Algorithms for the Diagnosis and Management of Musculoskeletal Complaints[6] and Institute for Clinical Systems Improvement[7]) include recommendations for non-pharmacological therapy, including patient education, social support, physical and occupational therapy, and exercise. In some of the guidelines, additional modalities recommended include weight loss, energy conservation, joint protection, heat, ice, acupuncture, massage and electrical stimulation. Pencharz *et al.* provide a critical appraisal of these sets of guidelines.[8] In a recent review of OA, pain management, patient education, psychological support, joint protection, exercise, goal-setting, assistive devices, heat/cold and weight reduction are recommended.[9]

PHYSICAL ACTIVITY AND EXERCISE

Physical activity has beneficial effects on cartilage health and, in theory, specific activity or exercise programmes may delay OA progression, although no evidence of this has been presented to date. It is also possible that certain activity or exercise programmes might *increase* the rate of OA progression. Several studies have examined the effect of recreational activity on incident OA, finding no deleterious effect, but little is known about the effect of specific activities on the risk of OA progression.

In general, the effect of strengthening exercise programmes on OA progression is unknown. In observational studies, the impact of strength differs: (1) between joint sites; (2) according to stage, i.e. whether the joint is relatively healthy, as in studies of incident OA, or arthritic, as in studies of OA progression; and (3) within a joint site, according to attributes of the local environment. In a study of incident OA, quadriceps strength protected against new development of knee OA in women.[10] In contrast to these findings for the knee, Chaisson *et al.* found that grip strength was associated with an increased risk of incident OA at the metacarpophalangeal (MCP) joints in women, and the proximal interphalangeal joints, MCP joints and thumb base in men.[11] Brandt *et al.* found no difference in baseline quadriceps strength between those who progressed and those who did not.[12] Similarly, we found no significant effect of strength on progression in OA knees considered as a whole.[13] However, in malaligned knees and in high-laxity knees, strength increased the likelihood of tibiofemoral OA progression. In more neutral or more stable knees, strength had neither a protective nor a deleterious effect.[13] These results suggest that in certain joint environments (e.g. malalignment or laxity), greater strength may translate into damaging joint forces. The strength/progression relationship in OA may differ according to these factors. Subset-specific approaches beyond strengthening exercise should be developed to enhance joint-protective muscle activity.

It is well-documented that regular physical activity and exercise benefit symptoms, function and quality of life, and they are critical components of OA management. Exercise for OA should address range of motion, flexibility, aerobic conditioning and muscle function. Muscle performance can be enhanced not only by strengthening exercise, but also by functional exercise to improve muscle endurance and motor control. The daily exercise regimen – in particular, exercises targeting range of motion and muscle function – should take into consideration the local joint pathology and impairments. In theory, exercise and activity benefits on pain and function in OA may be mediated through a variety of routes, including improvement in strength and endurance, cardiovascular fitness, self-efficacy and reduction in excess body weight and symptoms of depression or anxiety.

The American Geriatric Society Panel on Exercise and Osteoarthritis recently published consensus recommendations for exercise for older adults.[14] This is an evidenced-based review that delineates why a physically active lifestyle is beneficial to older adults with OA, and provides practical strategies and exercise guidelines for this population.

Van Baar et al. systematically reviewed exercise trials in patients with knee or hip OA.[15] In the six trials that met power and validity criteria, short-term benefits on pain and function were evident. There is less information about the long-term effects of exercise. In the 18-month FAST (Fitness, Arthritis and Seniors Trial), Ettinger et al. found that subjects with knee OA had modest improvement in measures of disability, physical performance and pain from participating in either an aerobic or a resistance exercise programme.[16] The reviews of Van Baar et al. and Baker and McAlindon[17] suggest that the effect sizes from studies of isolated strengthening exercise are lower than those from studies of more comprehensive interventions that include aerobic exercise, pain modalities and education.

In a recent randomized trial, Fransen et al. found a moderate effect of either individual or group physical therapy intervention (both including aerobic and strengthening components) compared with usual care on pain, physical function and health-related quality of life.[18] Baker et al. tested the effect of a high-intensity, home-based, progressive strength training programme and found significant improvement in WOMAC pain, WOMAC physical function, and self efficacy compared with a control group receiving a nutrition education programme.[19]

In their review, O'Reilly and Doherty note that minimal information is available on the effect of exercise on joint structure and, given experimental evidence to support both beneficial and detrimental effects of exercise on cartilage, more studies in this area are needed.[20] They also note that a combination of strengthening and aerobic exercise is, at present, the most practical approach, though little formal evaluation of type or intensity of either form of exercise has been undertaken. The question of whether exercise should be supervised or unsupervised has not been adequately studied. At present, the most practical approach is a gradual transition into a more unsupervised programme, with some maintenance of contact, as adherence is more likely to be lost without contact. Potentially important factors in adherence to exercise programmes include self-efficacy, previous exercise experience, baseline physical condition, peer and family support, disease severity and perception of benefit (Table 5.2).[20,21]

Rejeski *et al.* found that in subjects with knee pain and some difficulty with daily activity, there was a significant interaction of baseline self-efficacy with baseline knee strength in predicting both self-reported disability and stair-climb performance.[22] This adds support to the need to develop and test multifaceted approaches.

The beneficial effects of exercise decline with the passage of time from the period of an exercise intervention. Van Baar and colleagues randomized 201 subjects with hip or knee OA to either usual care or usual care plus supervised exercise for 12 weeks.[23] At 24 weeks, exercise treatment was associated with a small to moderate effect on pain during the past week; at 36 weeks, no differences were found between groups. These authors also summarize the limitations of prior studies, including the absence of an intention-to-treat analysis, high loss to follow-up, and combined data presentation for subjects with different types of arthritis. Most exercise trials have paid minimal attention to examining residual effects of exercise. Approaches to maximize long-term benefit include introduction of re-training or booster training, and steps to facilitate the acceptance of exercise and its practice.[23]

Table 5.2 Factors influencing adherence to exercise

Self-efficacy

Previous exercise experience

Baseline physical condition

Peer support

Family support

Disease severity

Co-morbidity

Perception of benefit

WEIGHT LOSS

There is strong epidemiologic evidence of the important role of body weight in the development of knee OA. Less is known about the impact of body weight on OA progression. In the Framingham study, weight in subjects of median age 37 years predicted the presence of knee OA 36 years later.[24] In Framingham women, a decrease in BMI of 2 units over the previous 10 years decreased the odds of knee OA (OR 0.46; 95% CI: 0.24, 0.86).[25] Higher BMI increased the risk of OA (OR 1.6/5 unit increase) in women, and weight change was directly correlated with the risk of OA (OR 1.4/10 lb change in weight).[26]

In a longitudinal study of the Chingford population (women; mean age 54 years), belonging to the top BMI tertile was associated with an increased risk of knee OA (OR 2.38, 95% CI: 1.29, 4.39).[27] In Chingford subjects with unilateral knee OA, 46% in the top BMI tertile developed OA in the uninvolved knee over 2 years versus 10% in the lowest tertile.[28]

The number of therapeutic trials examining the effect of weight loss in knee OA is relatively small. Knee pain was found in 14% of subjects after gastric stapling (and a mean weight loss of 45 kg) compared with 54% of subjects prior to this procedure.[29] Messier *et al.* compared exercise/weight reduction with exercise alone in older subjects with knee OA, and found that both groups lost weight and had significant improvement in pain and disability.[30] Huang *et al.* found that patients with knee OA and obesity who received a weight reduction intervention (including weekly auricular acupuncture, diet control and aerobic exercise), with or without ultrasound and transcutaneous electric stimulation treatment, had greater pain reduction, weight reduction, speed of ambulation and improvement in Lequesne index than patients who received only ultrasound and transcutaneous electric stimulation (Figure 5.1).[31]

NUTRITIONAL PRODUCTS

Several nutritional products are available that are touted as being beneficial for OA, but few have undergone rigorous testing. Among these, glucosamine and chondroitin sulphate have been evaluated in clinical trials, most of which received some manufacturer support. A meta-analysis suggested efficacy for symptoms, but also described evidence of publication bias, suggesting that the magnitude of the beneficial effect may be less than that reported.[32] Studies of glucosamine published since the meta-analysis have had mixed results, with some trials suggesting no or very modest difference between treatment and

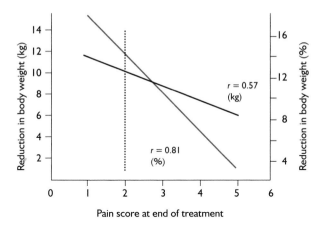

Figure 5.1 Regression lines for the correlation between change in body weight and pain score (mm on visual analogue scale (VAS)) and between change in body weight (%) and pain score (from the study by Huang *et al.*[31]). If weight reduction was more than 15%, a tolerable level of knee pain (< 2) was achieved

placebo (Figure 5.2).[33–35] The findings of Reginster *et al.* suggest some benefit of glucosamine on symptoms, albeit modest, even after 3 years of treatment,[36] and possibly a delay in radiographic progression. An NIH-funded, multicentre trial of glucosamine and chondroitin is ongoing.

In the Framingham study, dietary intake of vitamins C and D each appeared to protect against knee OA progression (but not incidence),[37,38] and a greater serum level of vitamin D appeared to protect against hip OA incidence.[39] Data are insufficient at present to support a therapeutic dose of vitamins C or D for the prevention or treatment of OA.[40] Although further research is necessary, it is advised that individuals with OA follow general public health recommendations by increasing their daily consumption of fruits and vegetables and optimizing their vitamin D status.[40]

EDUCATION

Patient education is recommended for the management of OA. OA patient education may have a specific focus, e.g. relaxation, cognitive pain management or exercise, or may be a multi-component programme. In a meta-analysis, pure instructional interventions were associated with relatively small effect sizes for

(a) Forest plot of effect sizes for trials and pooled effects

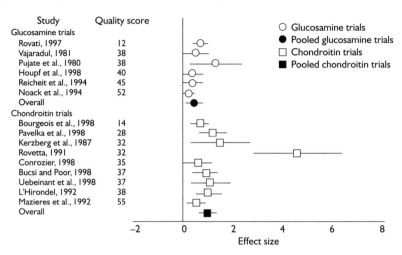

(b) Funnel plot of glucosamine and chondroitin trials

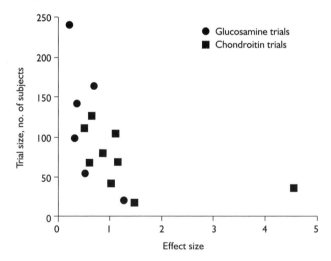

Figure 5.2 (a) The results (McAlindon *et al.*[32]) of the meta-analysis of glucosamine and chondroitin trials. Lines extending from the symbols represent 95% confidence intervals. A large effect size is suggested by 0.8, a moderate effect by 0.5, and a small effect by 0.2. (b) Funnel plots (McAlindon *et al.*[32]) developed from the meta-analysis. Both plots reveal asymmetry, suggesting the absence of trials with small numbers, and small or no treatment effect

outcomes of pain and disability, when compared with studies that had behavioural or psychological components (Figure 5.3).[41] Subsequently, Mazzuca *et al.* found in an attention-controlled clinical trial that the education group had significantly better disability and pain scores, though the former waned by 12 months.[42] Keefe and colleagues demonstrated that spouse-assisted coping skills training led to an improvement in coping, self-efficacy and physical disability compared with arthritis education-spousal support.[43] Hopman-Rock and Westhoff found that a self-management programme (health education and exercise instruction) for patients with knee or hip OA led to an improvement in mobility and pain compared with a control group receiving usual care.[44]

The Arthritis Self-Management Program (ASMP), taught in the community by trained lay leaders at weekly sessions, includes patient education on disease

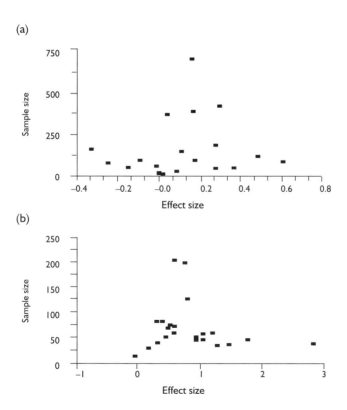

Figure 5.3 Plot of sample sizes versus effect sizes for pain in patient education studies (a) and non-steroidal anti-inflammatory drug (NSAID) studies (b)

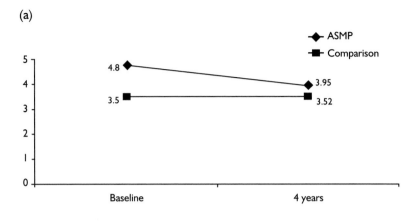

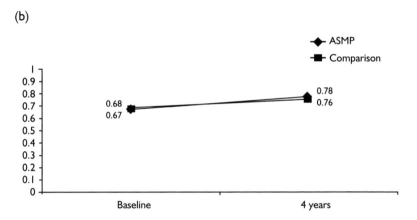

Figure 5.4 Mean baseline values and 4-year changes in health status among patients with osteoarthritis. (a) Pain; (b) disability. ASMP, The Arthritis Self-Management Program

processes, medication side-effects, exercise and cognitive-behavioural techniques, as well as a communication exercise in which participants learn to elicit support from family and friends.[45] The ASMP has been found to lead to improvements in: physical activity, use of cognitive pain-management techniques, pain;[45] long-term retention of initial gains (Figure 5.4);[46] use of self-management behaviours, such as exercise, communication with physicians, psychological well being;[47–49] knowledge, self-care behaviours, perceived helplessness and pain in individuals living in rural areas;[50] and knowledge, exercise, use of assistive devices and attitude in inner-city, low-literacy participants.[51] A major mechanism of the beneficial effect of the ASMP is enhanced self-efficacy.

ASMP sessions are now sponsored and/or organized by national voluntary arthritis organizations in the US, Canada and the UK, and use of the ASMP has also spread to Australia and New Zealand.

LATERAL-WEDGE INSOLES, FOOTWEAR AND BRACING FOR MEDIAL TIBIOFEMORAL OSTEOARTHRITIS

Varus alignment substantially increases the likelihood of progression of subsequent medial tibiofemoral OA.[3] For years, wedge osteotomy has been undertaken with the goal of reducing forces in the medial compartment in varus knees. Conservative approaches have also emerged. The use of a lateral-wedge insole is believed to lower medial compartment load and reduce lateral tensile forces by enhancing valgus correction of the calcaneus, whether or not varus deformity at the knee is lessened. This treatment has been shown in small, often uncontrolled trials to alleviate symptoms in medial compartment knee OA with varus alignment. Toda et al. theorized that talar motion may prevent calcaneal valgus correction, and examined the effect of a lateral-wedge insole with elastic strapping of the subtalar joint.[52] Participants wearing the strapped insole had significantly decreased femorotibial angle, talar tilt angle and pain (VAS); these differences were not found in the group with the traditional (unstrapped) insole. Adverse effects were more common in the strapped group (13%, e.g. popliteal pain, low-back pain, foot-sole pain) than in the traditional insert group (2%, foot-sole pain).

Maillefert et al. compared the effects of lateral-wedge insoles and neutral-wedge insoles (as control) in patients with medial knee OA, and found no difference between groups in the percentages of patients with improvement in WOMAC pain, stiffness or physical function scale scores.[53] The number of days of non-steroid anti-inflammatory drug intake during the preceding 3 months was significantly decreased at month 6 compared with baseline in the lateral-wedge insole group, whereas it remained unchanged in the other group.

Kerrigan and colleagues have found that wearing high-heel shoes leads to increases in forces across the medial and patellofemoral compartments.[54] Although the long-term effects of this type of footwear have not been elucidated, it seems prudent to minimize the wearing of high-heel shoes.

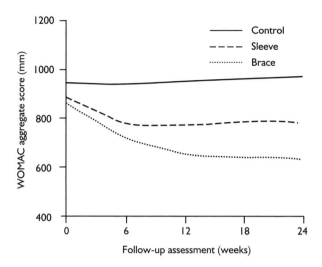

Figure 5.5 Kirkley *et al.*[56] found a significant difference between the unloader-brace group and the control group ($p < 0.001$), and a trend toward a difference between the brace group and the neoprene-sleeve group ($p = 0.06$), as well as between the neoprene-sleeve group and the control group ($p = 0.07$)

The goal of the valgus 'unloading' brace in medial knee OA is to produce an abduction moment to shift the joint contact force away from the stressed medial compartment. Matsuno *et al.* examined a series of 20 patients with mild to moderate knee OA treated with a Generation II knee brace, and found improvement in pain with walking and stairs, increased quadriceps strength and a small diminution in the severity of varus malalignment.[55] Kirkley *et al.* randomized subjects to: usual medical care; usual medical care plus a neoprene sleeve for the knee; or usual medical care plus an unloader brace.[56] At 6 months, the brace group had significantly better WOMAC scores (aggregate and pain scale) than the control group. Improvement over the neoprene-sleeve group was significant for the pain outcome and approached significance for the physical function outcomes (Figure 5.5). Groups did not differ in 6-minute walking test performance or stair-climbing test performance, although pain after these tasks was better in the bracing group.

The benefit of the neoprene sleeve in the trial by Kirkley *et al.* may reflect an improvement in proprioception. A number of small studies have shown that proprioception can be enhanced through the use of orthotics or exercise.

THERAPEUTIC ULTRASOUND, ACUPUNCTURE AND PULSED ELECTROMAGNETIC FIELD THERAPY

Pulsed ultrasound has been recommended for acute pain and inflammation, and continuous ultrasound for the treatment of restricted movement. Two meta-analyses concluded that there is poor evidence to support either the use or non-use of therapeutic ultrasound in the treatment of a variety of musculoskeletal conditions for pain control.[57,58] Puett and Griffin also found no literature support for ultrasound treatment prior to therapeutic exercise in the management of knee pain.[59] A recent Cochrane review,[60] including three studies, and among these, only one of high quality,[61] found no benefit over placebo or short-wave diathermy for patients with knee OA for pain relief, range of motion or functional status. Another Cochrane review, including one randomized controlled trial, found insufficient evidence for the inclusion of ultrasound in the treatment of patellofemoral pain syndrome.[62] For a more definitive answer on the use of therapeutic ultrasound in OA and patellofemoral pain, large, well-designed trials will be necessary.

Acupuncture has been more commonly applied for the treatment of OA symptoms in Asian countries, and has been the focus of several smaller studies. A systematic review in 1997 found inconsistent results and methodological flaws; the most rigorous studies suggested that acupuncture is not superior to sham treatment for OA pain.[63] In a follow-up study to a trial reported in 1999, Singh and colleagues found that a number of factors (including gender, race, age, Kellgren and Lawrence radiographic grade, obesity, knee tenderness, knee swelling, knee pain, knee crepitus) were not predictive of response to acupuncture treatment.[64,65] In a randomized, placebo-controlled, double-blind trial, Fink et al. found no difference in any outcomes (pain, function, activities of daily living, satisfaction) between the group receiving traditional acupuncture and the group receiving sham treatment (i.e. needles placed away from classic positions and not manipulated); the two groups showed comparable improvement.[66]

Pulsed electromagnetic field therapy, considered to be a remedy for delayed union fractures, has also been suggested as an alternative treatment for OA. Physical stress on bone leads to the appearance of piezoelectric potentials that may act as the transduction signals that promote bone formation; a similar mechanism exists in cartilage, in which chondrocytes are stimulated to increase proteoglycan synthesis. In a recent Cochrane review, only three studies were included.[67] Electrical stimulation therapy had a small to moderate effect on outcomes for knee OA, all statistically significant, with clinical benefit 13–23%

greater with active treatment compared with placebo. This therapy appeared to be less effective for cervical spine OA, with modest relative improvements in pain score (7.8%) and joint pain on motion (12%). Only one outcome for knee OA was clinically important (exceeding 20%). These findings demonstrate the need for larger studies to examine whether the statistically significant results translate into clinically important benefits.

Recently, Pipitone and Scott found that in 75 patients with knee OA by ACR criteria, in a double-blind, placebo-controlled randomized trial of 6 weeks' duration, there was no significant difference between active and sham treatment groups in pain reduction, WOMAC score or EuroQol score.[68] Paired analysis of follow-up observations on each patient showed significant improvements in the actively treated group (but not in the control group) in WOMAC overall score, WOMAC physical function and EuroQol score at study end, compared with baseline.

References

1. Lawrence RC, Helmick CG, Arnett FC, et al. Estimates of the prevalence of arthritis and selected musculoskeletal disorders in the United States. Arthritis Rheum 1998; 41: 778–99

2. Sharma L, Cahue S, Song J, et al. Physical functioning over 3 years in knee osteoarthritis: role of psychosocial, local mechanical and neuromuscular factors. Arthritis Rheum 2003; 48: 3359–70

3. Sharma L, Song J, Felson DT, et al. The role of knee alignment in disease progression and functional decline in knee osteoarthritis. J Am Med Assoc 2001; 286: 188–95

4. Altman RD, Hochberg MC, Moskowitz RW, Schnitzer TJ. Recommendations for the medical management of osteoarthritis of the hip and knee: 2000 update. Arthritis Rheum 2000; 43: 1905–15

5. Pendleton A, Arden N, Dougados M, et al. EULAR recommendations for the management of knee osteoarthritis: report of a task force of the Standing Committee for International Clinical Studies Including Therapeutic Trials (ESCISIT). Ann Rheum Dis 2000; 59: 936–44

6. Algorithms for the diagnosis and management of musculoskeletal complaints. Am J Med 1997; 103: 3S–6S

7. Lee JA. Adult degenerative joint disease of the knee: maximizing function and promoting joint health: Institute for Clinical System Integration. Postgrad Med 1999; 105: 183–97

8.   Pencharz JN, Grigoriadis E, Jansz GF, Bombardier C. A critical appraisal of clinical practice guidelines for the treatment of lower-limb osteoarthritis. Arthritis Res 2002; 4: 36–44

9.   McCarberg BH, Herr KA. Osteoarthritis: how to manage pain and improve patient function. Geriatrics 2001; 56: 14–24

10. Slemenda C, Heilman DK, Brandt KD, et al. Reduced quadriceps strength relative to body weight: a risk factor for knee osteoarthritis in women? Arthritis Rheum 1998; 41: 1951–9

11. Chaisson CE, Zhang Y, Sharma L, et al. Grip strength and the risk of developing radiographic hand osteoarthritis: results from the Framingham study. Arthritis Rheum 1999; 42: 33–8

12. Brandt KD, Heilman DK, Slemenda C, et al. Quadriceps strength in women with radiographically progressive osteoarthritis of the knee and those with stable radiographic changes. J Rheumatol 1999; 26: 2431–7

13. Sharma L, Dunlop DD, Cahue S, et al. Quadriceps strength and osteoarthritis progression in malaligned and lax knees. Ann Internal Med 2003; 138: 613–19

14. American Geriatric Society. Exercise prescription for older adults with osteoarthritis pain: consensus practice recommendations. J Am Geriatr Soc 2001; 49: 808–23

15. van Baar ME, Assendelft WJJ, Dekker J, et al. The effectiveness of exercise therapy in patients with osteoarthritis of the hip or knee. Arthritis Rheum 1999; 42: 1361–9

16. Ettinger WH, Burns R, Messier SP, et al. A randomized trial comparing aerobic exercise and resistance exercise with a health education program in older adults with knee osteoarthritis: the fitness arthritis and seniors trial. J Am Med Assoc 1997; 277: 25–31

17. Baker K, McAlindon T. Exercise for knee osteoarthritis. Curr Opin Rheumatol 2000; 12: 456–63

18. Fransen M, Crosbie J, Edmonds J. Physical therapy is effective for patients with osteoarthritis of the knee: a randomized controlled clinical trial. J Rheumatol 2001; 28: 156–64

19. Baker KR, Nelson ME, Felson DT, et al. The efficacy of home based progressive strength training in older adults with knee osteoarthritis: a randomized controlled trial. J Rheumatol 2001; 28: 1655–65

20. O'Reilly S, Doherty M. Lifestyle changes in the management of osteoarthritis. Best Pract Res Clin Rheumatol 2001; 15: 559–68

21. Rhodes RE, Martin AD, Taunton JE, et al. Factors associated with exercise adherence among older adults. Sports Medicine 1999; 28: 397–411

22. Rejeski WJ, Miller ME, Foy C, et al. Self-efficacy and the progression of functional limitations and self-reported disability in older adults with knee pain. J Gerontol B Psychol Sci Soc Sci 2001; 56: S261–5

23. van Baar ME, Dekker J, Oostendorp RAB, et al. Effectiveness of exercise in patients with osteoarthritis of hip or knee: nine months' follow up. Ann Rheum Dis 2001; 60: 1123–30

24. Felson DT, Anderson JJ, Naimark A, et al. Obesity and knee osteoarthritis, the Framingham study. Ann Intern Med 1988; 109: 18–24

25. Felson DT, Zhang Y, Anthony JM, et al. Weight loss reduces the risk for symptomatic knee osteoarthritis in women: the Framingham study. Ann Intern Med 1992; 116: 535–9

26. Felson DT, Zhang Y, Hannan MT, et al. Risk factors for incident radiographic knee osteoarthritis in the elderly. Arthritis Rheum 1997; 40: 728–33

27. Hart DJ, Doyle DV, Spector TD. Incidence and risk factors for radiographic knee osteoarthritis in middle-aged women, the Chingford Study. Arthritis Rheum 1999; 42: 17–24

28. Spector TD, Hart DJ, Doyle DV. Incidence and progression of osteoarthritis in women with unilateral knee disease in the general population: the effect of obesity. Ann Rheum Dis 1994; 53: 565–8

29. McGoey BV, Deitel M, Saplys RJ, Kliman ME. Effect of weight loss on musculoskeletal pain in the morbidly obese. J Bone Joint Surg Br 1990; 72: 322–3

30. Messier SP, Loeser RF, Mitchell MN, et al. Exercise and weight loss in obese older adults with knee osteoarthritis: a preliminary study. J Am Geriatr Soc 2000; 48: 1072–2000

31. Huang MH, Chen CH, Chen TW, et al. The effects of weight reduction on the rehabilitation of patients with knee osteoarthritis and obesity. Arthritis Care Res 2000; 13: 398–405

32. McAlindon TE, LaValley MP, Gulin JP, Felson DT. Glucosamine and chondroitin for treatment of osteoarthritis; a systematic quality assessment and meta-analysis. J Am Med Assoc 2000; 283: 1469–75

33. Houpt JB, McMillan R, Wein C, Paget-Dellio SD. Effect of glucosamine hydrochloride in the treatment of pain of osteoarthritis of the knee. J Rheumatol 1999; 26: 2423–30

34. Hughes RA, Carr AJ. A randomized double-blind placebo-controlled trial of glucosamine to control pain in osteoarthritis of the knee. Arthritis Rheum 2000; 43: S384

35. Rindone JP, Hiller D, Collacott E, et al. Randomized, controlled trial of glucosamine for treating osteoarthritis of the knee. West J Med 2000; 172: 91–4

36. Reginster JY, Deroisy R, Rovati LC, et al. Long-term effects of glucosamine sulphate on osteoarthritis progression: a randomized, placebo-controlled clinical trial. Lancet 2001; 357: 251–6

37. McAlindon TE, Jacques P, Zhang Y, et al. Do antioxidant micronutrients protect against the development and progression of knee osteoarthritis? Arthritis Rheum 1996; 39: 648–56

38. McAlindon TE, Felson DT, Zhang Y, et al. Relation of dietary intake and serum levels of vitamin D to progression of osteoarthritis of the knee among participants in the Framingham Study. Ann Intern Med 1996; 125: 353–9

39. Lane NE, Gore LR, Cummings SR, et al. Serum vitamin D levels and incident changes of radiographic hip osteoarthritis: a longitudinal study. Study of Osteoporosis Fractures Research Group. Arthritis Rheum 1999; 42: 854–60

40. McAlindon TE. Mechanisms by which micronutrients may influence osteoarthritis. In Brandt KD, Doherty M, Lohamander S, eds. Osteoarthritis, 2nd edn. Oxford: Oxford University Press, 2003: 295

41. Superio-Cabuslay E, Ward M, Lorig K. Patient education interventions in osteoarthritis and rheumatoid arthritis: a meta-analytic comparison with nonsteroidal antiinflammatory drug treatment. Arthritis Care Res 1996; 9: 292–301

42. Mazzuca SA, Brandt KD, Katz BP, et al. Effects of self-care education on the health status of inner-city patients with osteoarthritis of the knee. Arthritis Rheum 1997; 40: 1466–74

43. Keefe FJ, Caldwell DS, Baucom D, et al. Spouse-assisted coping skills training in the management of osteoarthritis knee pain. Arthritis Care Res 1996; 9: 279–91

44. Hopman-Rock M, Westoff MH. The effects of a health education and exercise program for older adults with osteoarthritis of the hip or knee. J Rheumatol 2000; 27: 1947–54

45. Lorig K, Holman HR. Arthritis self-management studies: a 12 year review. Health Educ Q 1993; 20: 17–28

46. Lorig K, Mazonson P, Holman H. Evidence suggesting that health education for self-management in patients with chronic arthritis has sustained health benefits while reducing health care costs. Arthritis Rheum 1993; 36: 439–46

47. Barlow JH, Turner A, Wright CC. A randomized controlled study of the Arthritis Self Management Program in the UK. Health Educ Res 2000; 15: 665–80

48. Barlow JH, Williams B, Wright C. Instilling the strength to fight the pain and get on with life: learning to become an arthritis self-manager through an adult education program. Health Educ Res 1999; 14: 533–44

49. Barlow JH, Williams RG, Wright C. Improving arthritis self-management in older adults: just what the doctor didn't order. Br J Health Psychol 1997; 2: 175–85

50. Goeppinger J, Brunk SE, Arthur MW, Reidesel S. The effectiveness of community-based arthritis self-care programs. Arthritis Rheum 1987; 30: S194

51. Bill-Harvey D, Rippy R, Abeles M, et al. Outcome of an osteoarthritis education program for low-literacy patients taught by indigenous instructors. Patient Educ Counsel 1989; 13: 133–42

52. Toda Y, Segal N, Kato A, et al. Effect of a novel insole on the subtalar joint of patients with medial compartment osteoarthritis of the knee. J Rheumatol 2001; 28: 2705–10

53. Maillefert JF, Hudry C, Baron G, et al. Laterally elevated wedged insoles in the treatment of medial knee osteoarthritis: a prospective randomized controlled study. Osteoarthritis Cartilage 2001; 9: 738–45

54. Kerrigan DC, Todd MK, O'Riley PO. Knee osteoarthritis and high-heeled shoes. Lancet 1998; 351: 1399–1401

55. Matsuno H, Kadowaki KM, Tsuji H. Generations II knee bracing for severe medial compartment osteoarthritis of the knee. Arch Phys Med Rehabil 1997; 78: 745–9

56. Kirkley A, Webster-Bogaert S, Litchfield R, et al. The effect of bracing on varus gonarthrosis. J Bone Joint Surg Am 1999; 81: 539–48

57. van der Windt DAWM, van der Heijden GJ, van den Berg SGM, et al. Ultrasound for musculoskeletal disorders: a systematic review. Pain 1999; 81: 257–71

58. Gam AN, Johannsen F. Ultrasound therapy in musculoskeletal disorders: a meta-analysis. Pain 1995; 63: 85–91

59. Puett DW, Griffin MR. Published trials of nonmedicinal and noninvasive therapies for the hip and knee osteoarthritis. Ann Intern Med 1994; 121: 133–40

60. Welch V, Brosseau L, Peterson J, et al. Therapeutic ultrasound for osteoarthritis of the knee [Review]. Cochrane Database Syst Rev 2001: CD003132

61. Falconer J, Hayes KW, Chang RW. Effect of ultrasound on mobility in osteoarthritis of the knee. Arthritis Care Res 1992; 5: 29–35

62. Brosseau L, Casimiro L, Robinson V, et al. Therapeutic ultrasound for treating patellofemoral pain syndrome [Review]. Cochrane Database Syst Rev 2001: CD003375

63. Ernst E. Acupuncture as a symptomatic treatment of osteoarthritis. A systematic review. Scand J Rheumatol 1997; 26: 444–7

64. Berman BM, Singh BB, Lao L, et al. A randomized trial of acupuncture as an adjunctive therapy in osteoarthritis of the knee. Rheumatology (Oxford) 1999; 38: 346–54

65. Singh BB, Berman BM, Hadhazy V, et al. Clinical decisions in the use of acupuncture as an adjunctive therapy for osteoarthritis of the knee. Altern Ther Health Med 2001; 7: 58–65

66. Fink MG, Kunsebeck H, Wipperman B, Gehrke A. Non-specific effects of traditional Chinese acupuncture in osteoarthritis of the hip. Complement Ther Med 2001; 9: 82–8

67. Hulme J, Robinson V, DeBie R, et al. Electromagnetic fields for the treatment of osteoarthritis [Review]. Cochrane Database Syst Rev 2002: CD003523

68. Pipitone N, Scott DL. Magnetic pulse treatment for knee osteoarthritis: a randomised, double-blind, placebo-controlled study. Curr Med Res Opin 2001; 17: 190–6

6

Pharmacological treatments

Kelsey M Jordan, Nigel Arden

INTRODUCTION

Osteoarthritis (OA) is a common condition, associated with pain and functional disability. Physical disability resulting from pain and loss of functional capacity reduces quality of life and further increases the risk of morbidity and mortality. Current treatments aim to alleviate these symptoms by several different methods.

This chapter will review oral, topical and intra-articular treatments commonly used in patients with OA. The efficacy and safety profile of each treatment will be assessed and, where possible, its benefit quantified. Where practicable, the effect size (ES) has been calculated for pain as an outcome measure.[1] The ES reflects the standardized mean difference between the treatment and placebo groups. Clinically, an effect size of 0.2 is considered small, 0.5 is moderate (and would be recognized clinically) and greater than 0.8 is large (Table 6.1).

A treatment algorithm for the management of OA is presented, which advocates a step-wise increase in treatment depending on symptoms and functional impairment (Figure 6.1). It should be remembered that pharmacological treatments should always be combined with non-pharmacological treatments for optimum effect and tailored to the individual requirements of the patient.

Table 6.1 Effect size and level of evidence of pharmacological treatments

Intervention	Effect size (range)	Level of evidence
Paracetamol	*	1B
Conventional NSAIDs	0.47–0.96	1A
Coxib NSAIDs	0.5	1B
Opioid analgesics	*	1B
Topical NSAIDs	0–1.03	1A
Topical capsaicin	0.41–0.56	1A
Glucosamine sulphate	0.43–1.02	1A
Chondroitin sulphate	1.23–1.50	1A
Intra-articular corticosteroid	1.27	1A
Intra-articular hyaluronic acid	0–0.9	1B

*Unable to calculate; NSAID, non-steroidal anti-inflammatory drug

PARACETAMOL (ACETAMINOPHEN)

Background

Paracetamol was first used by von Mering in 1893,[2] but was not used commercially until the 1950s. Today, many patients use paracetamol bought over the counter or on prescription for mild to moderate pain; it has few serious interactions and is proposed to be a safe and effective medicine, particularly in the elderly. It has been estimated that 22% of the adult population in the US use paracetamol in any given week.[3]

The European League against Rheumatism (EULAR), in its updated recommendations, states that: 'Paracetamol is the oral analgesic of first choice and, if successful, the preferred long-term oral analgesic.'[4] Recommendations from the American College of Rheumatology (ACR) also state that paracetamol should be the first analgesic to be used for mild to moderate pain in OA, based on its overall cost, efficacy and toxicity profile.[5]

Safety profile

Paracetamol has a good safety record and has traditionally been regarded as having no serious side-effects. Recently, however, concerns about the safety of paracetamol were raised by an epidemiological study of 958 397 subjects in the UK, which suggested that high doses of paracetamol may convey the same excess

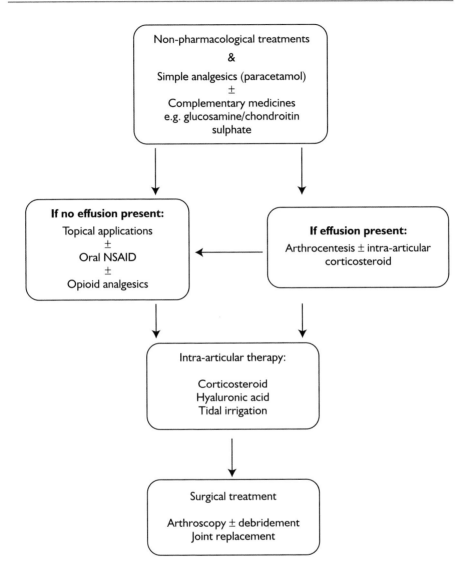

Figure 6.1 Algorithm for the use of pharmacological treatments in the management of osteoarthritis

risk of upper gastrointestinal (GI) complications as traditional non-steroidal anti-inflammatory drugs (NSAIDs). Although users of paracetamol at doses less than 2 g/day did not have an increased risk of GI complications, those taking over 2 g/day had an adjusted relative risk (RR) of GI complications of 3.6; this lies between the RR of 2.4 seen in low/medium-dose NSAID use and 4.9 in high-dose NSAID use.[6] This study, however, did not adjust for important co-morbid conditions, and therefore may have overestimated the risk of complications. The above finding is supported by a retrospective study of 26 978 subjects aged ≥ 65 years, which demonstrated that patients at a higher risk of GI adverse events were more likely to have been prescribed paracetamol than an NSAID. In this study, there was a dose-related increase in GI adverse events; however, these predominantly related to dyspepsia, rather than hospitalization, perforations, ulcers and bleeds.[7] Furthermore, an earlier report that surveyed 62 216 patients in California reported 1074 drug-related problems for all drugs. Of these, 77 had GI adverse events associated with aspirin or ibuprofen; the only GI problem associated with paracetamol was constipation, in 28 patients.[8] In summary, low-dose paracetamol appears to be a safe drug, but at higher doses may be associated with non-serious GI adverse events.

Issues of safety also arise when medicating patients with chronic premorbid conditions such as alcohol misuse and cirrhosis. Liver toxicity is well recognized in paracetamol overdose, but treatment of patients with OA who have cirrhosis or who misuse alcohol has triggered heated debate among physicians. Given that paracetamol use is so high (22%), and that alcohol misuse affects up to 10% of the population, one would be likely to see many reports of toxicity in this group of patients, should an adverse interaction exist. A prospective, double-blind, two-period crossover study gave 20 subjects with stable, chronic liver disease paracetamol 4000 mg/day for 13 days. No abnormalities indicative of an adverse reaction were seen.[9] In a randomized, double-blind, placebo-controlled study of 201 subjects, recruited from an alcohol detoxification centre, there were no differences in liver enzyme changes from baseline between the placebo and paracetamol 4000 mg/day groups. These reports would therefore negate the argument that paracetamol produces liver injury in alcoholic patients, and suggest that it is a safe analgesic to use.

What is the evidence?

Despite its historical use, there are few good-quality studies examining the efficacy of paracetamol. Most studies do not mimic how paracetamol is taken in the community, as they are conducted over short periods of time and include small numbers of participants; there is often no comparison with placebo. In one study – a 6-week cross-over, double-blind, randomized controlled trial (RCT) comparing 4 g/day of paracetamol with placebo in 25 subjects with knee OA – pain outcomes showed significant improvement with paracetamol.[10]

Paracetamol has, however, been compared with NSAIDs in a number of studies, with varying outcomes. A 4-week RCT compared paracetamol 4 g/day with ibuprofen 1200 mg/day and 2400 mg/day in 184 subjects. All outcomes were similar at the end of the trial between paracetamol and ibuprofen, with the exception of rest pain, which was better controlled in the NSAID group.[11] These data were re-evaluated almost 10 years later to investigate if severe disease would behave in a different manner to mild/moderate disease; this study demonstrated that even severe knee pain responded equally to paracetamol and ibuprofen.[12] A 2-year study compared paracetamol 2600 mg/day with naproxen 750 mg/day in 178 subjects with knee OA. The study examined both radiographic progression and withdrawal from the trial from lack of efficacy. There was a huge dropout over the 2 years in both arms of the trial (35%), due to lack of efficacy. At 6 weeks, the naproxen group had significant improvements in pain at rest, pain on motion, 50-foot walk time and doctor assessment, whereas those receiving paracetamol only had improvements in pain on motion and doctor assessment. At 2 years, however, the only difference between the two groups was improvement in the 50-foot walk in the naproxen group.[13]

A 12-week cross-over study compared paracetamol 4000 mg/day with diclofenac/misoprostol 150 mg/400 µg in 227 subjects with knee or hip OA. The NSAID resulted in significantly greater improvements in pain scores, although subjects with milder symptomatic and/or radiographic disease had similar improvements with both drugs; in this study, the paracetamol group had fewer adverse events.[14] Paracetamol 4000 mg/day has also been compared with both rofecoxib* (12.5 mg/day and 25 mg/day) and celecoxib 200 mg/day in 382 participants with knee OA in a 6-week study. Rofecoxib* 25 mg was significantly superior for night pain and a composite pain sub-score, compared with all other arms in the trial; adverse events were similar in all four groups.[15] More recently, a study from the US in 82 subjects compared paracetamol 4000 mg/day, placebo and diclofenac 150 mg/day;[16] only the patients in the diclofenac group had a significant improvement in WOMAC pain score at 2 and 12 weeks. The authors concluded that paracetamol was no better than placebo.

Patient preference

There is little information documenting which treatments patients prefer using. One study found that 57% of participants were more likely to report that an NSAID was better or much better than paracetamol.[14] In a further study, a 15-minute telephone survey was conducted with 300 patients.[17] Interestingly, most patients did not continue to take their drugs for more than 2 years; in those who did, paracetamol was the most commonly continued medication, and paracetamol was significantly less likely to be discontinued due to toxicity than NSAIDs. About 30% of patients taking paracetamol also took an NSAID.

Summary

A systematic review concluded that the evidence available to date supports the efficacy of both paracetamol and NSAIDs in the management of OA, and that NSAIDs are superior to paracetamol in terms of pain reduction and improvement in patients' and physicians' global assessments. No differences in terms of functional status were found. The benefits of NSAIDs over paracetamol were modest and the authors therefore suggested that other factors are also important in deciding which drugs to use to treat patients with OA. These factors include the patient's preference, the prescriber's clinical judgement, cost and comparative safety of the individual drugs.[18] It would therefore seem prudent to initiate treatment with paracetamol and add to it if pain is not adequately controlled.

NON-STEROIDAL ANTI-INFLAMMATORY DRUGS

Background

NSAIDs have been in use for hundreds of years. Hippocrates advocated willow bark for the treatment of pain and inflammation in ancient Greece. In more recent times, the first 'clinical trial' of aspirin was accredited to Dr Thomas MacLagan in 1876, who tried it on himself, and then in patients with acute rheumatism, resulting in complete remission of their symptoms. Ibuprofen was identified by the Boots Company in the early 1950s, and was in widespread use by the 1970s for treating musculoskeletal complaints.[19] Since then, multiple NSAIDs have been developed, and they are one of the most widely prescribed therapeutic agents. In recent years, NSAIDs that selectively inhibit cyclo-oxygenase 2 (COX-2) have been developed and offer the promise of efficacy without the GI toxicity seen with conventional NSAIDs.

Both EULAR and the ACR have recommended the use of NSAIDs in patients with pain unresponsive to paracetamol.[4,5] EULAR have also recommended: 'In patients with an increased gastrointestinal risk, non-selective

NSAIDs and effective gastro-protective agents, or selective COX-2 inhibitors, should be used.'

Safety profile

NSAIDs, as a class, are associated with an increase in upper GI serious (ulcers, bleeds and perforations) and nuisance (bloating, dyspepsia) complications, nephrotoxicity and cardiovascular adverse events.

Risk factors for upper GI complications include: age > 65 years, a history of peptic ulcer disease or upper GI bleed, concomitant use of oral anticoagulants or corticosteroids. Compared with non-users, the RR of developing serious upper GI complications with low/medium and high doses of conventional NSAIDs has been shown to be 2.4 and 4.9, respectively, demonstrating a doubling of risk in those taking full doses.[6] Upper GI symptoms are very common; overall, 15–40% of patients taking NSAIDs experience dyspepsia, and both non-aspirin NSAIDs and aspirin itself are independent risk factors for the development of dyspeptic symptoms.[20]

Given the increase in GI toxicity when using NSAIDs, there has been much interest in gastro-protective agents used in combination with NSAIDs to reduce this risk. A Cochrane review examined the effectiveness of interventions for the prevention of NSAID-induced upper GI toxicity, including 40 RCTs. The authors concluded that all doses of misoprostol significantly reduce the risk of endoscopic duodenal, but not gastric, ulcers and that double doses of histamine-2 receptor antagonists (H2RAs) and protein pump inhibitors (PPIs) effectively reduce the risk of endoscopic duodenal and gastric ulcers, and are better tolerated than misoprostol. It must be stressed, however, that the healing rate of these agents is 63% for H2RAs and 80% for PPIs; therefore, a proportion of patients will remain at risk of upper GI complications even when using gastro-protective agents.

The anti-inflammatory effects of non-selective NSAIDs appear to be mediated via COX-2 inhibition, while the harmful effects in the GI tract and on platelets are believed to occur primarily due to COX-1 inhibition. Therefore, COX-2 selective drugs should theoretically provide efficacy without the harmful GI effects and platelet dysfunction. Recent studies have demonstrated that COX-2 selective drugs reduce the risk of perforations, ulcers, bleeds and endoscopic ulcers by 50% or more,[21–23] compared with conventional NSAIDs, but with comparable efficacy. In a US population, it was found that celecoxib use was associated with a significantly decreased risk of outpatient physician claims for upper GI symptoms, compared with the commonly used prescription NSAIDs ibuprofen and naproxen.[24]

Both conventional and COX-2 selective NSAIDs have an effect on the cardiovascular system. In a retrospective study, NSAID-naive patients aged over 65 years were identified who were subsequently commenced on conventional NSAID ($n = 5391$), rofecoxib* ($n = 14\,583$) or celecoxib ($n = 18\,908$), and compared with controls ($n = 100\,000$) who had not taken an NSAID.[25] Relative to non-NSAID users, patients taking conventional NSAIDs and rofecoxib* had a higher risk of admission for congestive heart failure; those taking celecoxib had a similar risk. A long-term outcome study of 8538 patients found that patients taking rofecoxib* were significantly more likely to develop hypertension and peripheral oedema, compared with conventional NSAID or celecoxib users.[26] The full effects of NSAIDs on the cardiovascular system are still unknown, however, and many studies are inconclusive. Some studies suggest that naproxen may have a cardioprotective effect, similar to low-dose aspirin. Other studies have suggested that COX-2 selective drugs may have a variety of beneficial cardiovascular effects – on endothelial function, and reducing low-grade inflammation and oxidative stress in patients with severe coronary heart disease and, in combination with aspirin, improving clinical symptoms.[27] Further large studies are required to explore these findings. There is no doubt that all NSAIDs (including COX-2 selective drugs) can potentially cause ankle oedema and an increase in blood pressure in susceptible individuals.

What is the evidence?

Two Cochrane reviews have investigated the use of conventional NSAIDs for hip and knee OA.[28,29] Their conclusion was that, despite the large number of trials performed, the quality was often poor and there were few randomized placebo-controlled trials. All the drugs studied were more efficacious than placebo, but there were few discernible differences between them at standard dosages (etodolac, naproxen, diclofenac, indomethacin, piroxicam, sulindac and nabumetone). Drugs used at low dose (ibuprofen and naproxen) were found to be lower risk, and indomethacin was found to be the most toxic of the drugs studied. The authors suggested that the selection of an NSAID should be based upon relative safety, patient acceptability and cost.

With the advent of the COX-2 selective NSAIDs, the general quality of study design has improved enormously. Celecoxib and rofecoxib* have been investigated in robust RCTs, demonstrating equivalent efficacy to conventional

NSAIDs. Rofecoxib* has shown clinical efficacy comparable to that of high-dose ibuprofen[30,31] and diclofenac.[32] Celecoxib has shown comparable efficacy to naproxen[33] and diclofenac.[34] These drugs are all significantly superior to placebo.

Most of the NSAID studies have been of short duration, generally over 6–12 weeks. Few studies have examined their effects for longer periods of time. Studies that have explored the use of NSAIDs for 6 months or longer[31,32,35–37] demonstrate drop-out rates of 35–50%, primarily due to the onset of adverse events, making interpretation of the results somewhat difficult. A study investigating the long-term efficacy of two NSAIDs demonstrated significant reductions in pain, compared with placebo, at 4 weeks, but pain scores similar to placebo between 1 and 3 years later, with the majority of OA patients experiencing pain and disability despite therapy.

Summary

There is no doubt that NSAIDs – both conventional and COX-2 specific – are efficacious in providing short-term pain relief to patients with OA. There is, however, concern over their safety, particularly with regard to upper GI complications. Gastro-protective agents or COX-2 selective agents can be used to reduce these risks, but a proportion of patients will always be susceptible.

TOPICAL NON-STEROIDAL ANTI-INFLAMMATORY DRUGS

Background

Patients with OA and other musculoskeletal conditions often use topical NSAIDs. They are a common prescription medication and are also readily available as over-the-counter medications, and are well tolerated and safe to use. Topical NSAIDs can provide an effective alternative for the management of pain by delivering the drug locally, without the GI complications encountered with many oral NSAIDs.

Despite good evidence from several well-designed placebo-controlled studies and a systematic review supporting their efficacy, there is often a scientifically unfounded view within the medical community that it is merely the 'rubbing in' of the topical application that produces an effect!

Safety profile

Topical NSAIDs have a good safety record. Indeed, a large surveillance study, performed in general practice, suggested good safety (adverse events < 1.5%), with local skin reactions being the main adverse effect.[38] A large case–control study of 320 000 people in Scotland found that 7% had been prescribed a topical NSAID and that there was never an association with upper GI bleeding and/or perforation, irrespective of the control population used or the duration of use of the topical NSAID.[39] Individual placebo-controlled RCTs would further support these findings. A systematic review of topical NSAIDs used in chronic conditions, in particular OA, found few local or systemic adverse events, and certainly no differences from placebo.[40]

What is the evidence?

The systematic review assessed the efficacy of topically applied NSAID in reducing pain to at least half its baseline level at 2 weeks; 13 placebo-controlled trials were included, with 547 patients in the active-treatment arm and 550 treated with placebo. Topical NSAID was significantly superior in reducing pain; 65% of patients treated with topical NSAID at least halved their pain scores, compared with 30% treated with placebo. The number of patients needed to treat to get one improvement was 3.1.[40] More recent blinded, randomized studies assessing the benefit of topical NSAIDs for the treatment of knee OA found that eltenac gel was significantly better than placebo in patients with severe OA, but not mild to moderate OA,[41] whereas diclofenac gel was significantly better than placebo in patients with mild to moderate OA.[42] A different study showed equivalent benefit with piroxicam gel versus a homeopathic gel in 172 patients.[43]

TOPICAL CAPSAICIN

Background

Capsaicin, the most pungent ingredient in red chilli peppers, has been used for centuries to remedy pain. Capsaicin reversibly desensitizes nociceptive C fibres by acting on VR-1 vaniloid receptors. First exposure to capsaicin intensely activates these fibres (orthodromic: pain sensation; antidromic: local reddening, oedema, etc.). After the first exposure, the sensory neurons become insensitive to all further stimulation (including capsaicin itself). In order to be optimally effective, topical capsaicin must be applied repeatedly (3–4 times daily) on the painful area to obtain desensitization. Capsaicin has also been used successfully in controlling neuropathic pain, in particular in postherpetic neuralgia and diabetic neuropathy.

Safety profile

Capsaicin may be an irritant to the skin, particularly during the first few days of use, and patients should be counselled accordingly. The irritant effect is generally self-limiting. Handling may produce a contact dermatitis. No systemic side-effects have been reported.

What is the evidence?

There are few good-quality studies examining the effects of topical capsaicin on OA. One controlled study found that capsaicin was significantly superior to placebo in reducing knee OA pain, which was sustained at 4 weeks;[44] another study demonstrated a significant decrease in tenderness and pain in patients with hand OA.[45] More recently, both capsaicin and glyceryl trinitrate have been found to have an analgesic effect superior to that of placebo in patients with OA and, when used concomitantly, it would appear they have an additive effect.[46]

Summary

Topical applications are efficacious and safe. They can be used as an 'add-on' therapy to simple analgesics, or as an alternative in those who are unable to tolerate oral analgesics and NSAIDs, or if these medications are contraindicated.

INTRA-ARTICULAR CORTICOSTEROID

Background

Intra-articular corticosteroid injections were first used in the early 1950s to obviate the need for systemic corticosteroids. The inflammatory arthritides are the most frequently met conditions treated in this manner. Flares of pain, due to OA, particularly affecting the knee (with or without effusion) and hand, have also been shown to improve following corticosteroid injection. It would appear that a change in the inflammatory process occurs, which persists after the corticosteroid has left the joint. Patients are advised to rest the injected joint for 24–48 hours following the procedure, in order to minimize leakage and improve the anti-inflammatory response. A controlled study of 24-hours' rest following knee injection enhanced the benefits, which persisted up to 6 months.[47]

There has been speculation that repeated injection may promote joint destruction and tissue atrophy. Recent evidence has proven that repeated intra-articular corticosteroid injection performed every 3 months over a 2-year period has no long-term deleterious effects on the anatomical structure of the knee, and may even be an effective alternative treatment in those who are unable to undergo a surgical procedure by alleviating pain.[48]

Safety profile

There are few absolute contraindications to joint injection (Figure 6.2). The presence of a bleeding diathesis, anticoagulation or overlying skin infection or

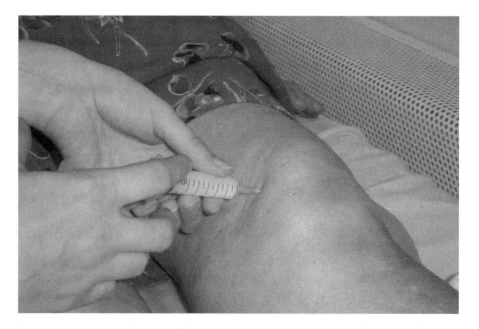

Figure 6.2 Intra-articular knee injection. A medial, infra-patellar, straight-leg approach

Table 6.2 Potential complications and side-effects of intra-articular injections

Complication	Contraindication (relative)
Septic arthritis	Overlying skin disease or infection
Skin/fat atrophy	Significant bleeding diathesis
Skin/fat depigmentation	Anticoagulation
Misplaced injection	Prosthetic joint
Tendon rupture	Systemic infection
Nerve damage	
Local extravasation	

systemic infection may preclude injection (Table 6.2). Septic arthritis is the most important complication, and has been estimated to occur in less than 1 : 14 000 procedures.[49] However, given the serious medical implications of septic arthritis, all patients must be made aware of this potential risk. No serious adverse events were reported in any clinical trials conducted, though a small number of participants developed transient local discomfort.

What is the evidence?

A recent meta-analysis pooled ten RCTs to ascertain the effects of intra-articular corticosteroid on knee OA. A significant improvement in symptoms was seen in the active-treatment groups. The RR for improvement up to 2 weeks after injection was 1.66, and the number needed to treat to get one improvement was 1.3–3.5 patients (Figure 6.3a). In the higher-quality studies, improvement could be assessed over a longer time period (16–24 weeks); the pooled results gave a RR of 2.09 and a number needed to be treated of 4.4 (Figure 6.3b). Varying doses of corticosteroid were used (the equivalent of 6.25–80 mg prednisolone). Those studies showing benefit for a longer duration used higher doses of corticosteroid (the equivalent of 50 mg prednisolone).[50]

Unfortunately, predictors of response to corticosteroid injection are unclear. Conflicting results have been obtained with regard to the presence of a joint effusion. One randomized controlled study of 84 patients confirmed a short-term benefit of steroid over placebo, with a better outcome in those with an effusion.[51] However, a randomized cross-over study of methylprednisolone

(a)

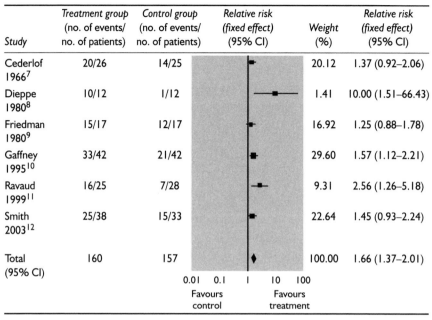

Study	Treatment group (no. of events/ no. of patients)	Control group (no. of events/ no. of patients)	Relative risk (fixed effect) (95% CI)	Weight (%)	Relative risk (fixed effect) (95% CI)
Cederlof 1966[7]	20/26	14/25		20.12	1.37 (0.92–2.06)
Dieppe 1980[8]	10/12	1/12		1.41	10.00 (1.51–66.43)
Friedman 1980[9]	15/17	12/17		16.92	1.25 (0.88–1.78)
Gaffney 1995[10]	33/42	21/42		29.60	1.57 (1.12–2.21)
Ravaud 1999[11]	16/25	7/28		9.31	2.56 (1.26–5.18)
Smith 2003[12]	25/38	15/33		22.64	1.45 (0.93–2.24)
Total (95% CI)	160	157		100.00	1.66 (1.37–2.01)

0.01   0.1   1   10   100

Favours control   Favours treatment

Test for heterogeneity $\chi^2 = 8.70$, df = 5, $p = 0.12$, $p = 42.5\%$
Test for overall effect $z = 5.14$, $p < 0.00001$

(b)

Study	Treatment group (no. of events/ no. of patients)	Control group (no. of events/ no. of patients)	Relative risk (fixed effect) (95% CI)	Weight (%)	Relative risk (fixed effect) (95% CI)
Ravaud 1999[11]	12/25	6/28		43.0	2.24 (0.99–5.08)
Smith 2003[12]	16/38	7/33		57.0	1.98 (0.93–4.23)
Total (95% CI)	28/63	13/61		100.00	2.09 (1.20–3.65)

0.1 0.2   1   5   10

Favours control   Favours treatment

Test for heterogeneity $\chi^2 = 0.05$, df = 1, $p = 0.83$
Test for overall effect $z = 2.61$, $p = 0.009$

Figure 6.3 (a) Improvements up to 2 weeks after corticosteroid injection into the knee. (b) Improvements 16–24 weeks after high-dose corticosteroid injection into the knee

versus saline found no clinical predictors of response, suggesting that corticosteroid should not be reserved only for those with effusion.[52]

Summary

Intra-articular corticosteroid injections are highly efficacious in relieving the symptoms of knee OA for at least a 1–4-week period. Higher doses may achieve a longer duration of effect. There is no evidence that repeated injection damages the joint in any way, which is of benefit to those patients who are too brittle to undergo a surgical procedure. The evidence for predictors of response, however, remains unclear, and further studies are required to answer this question.

INTRA-ARTICULAR HYALURONIC ACID

Background

Hyaluronans (HAs) were first developed in the 1960s by Balazs.[53] HA is a large glycosaminoglycan composed of repeating disaccharides, which is found in the cartilage matrix. HA has both viscous and elastic properties, acting as an elastic shock absorber and storing energy during rapid joint movements and dissipating energy by acting as a viscous lubricant during slow movements. HA has been postulated to protect the joints by acting in this way. HA is diminished in OA, with a reduction in both its concentration and molecular weight.[54] It has been speculated that replacement of HA in patients with OA, to restore the healthy synovial fluid balance of the joint, may be efficacious in terms of pain relief and physical function. Many trials have attempted to address this question, often with conflicting results. As with the intra-articular corticosteroid studies, patient predictors of response to treatment have not been identified, although those HAs with a higher molecular weight have been suggested to be more efficacious.

Controversy also continues about the potential disease-modifying effects of HA compounds on OA. Animal models have provided conflicting reports. Arthroscopic studies in human subjects recruited a low number of participants, but did potentially demonstrate a disease-modifying effect of HA in slowing the progression of chondropathy following intra-articular HA injection. These studies need to be repeated in larger numbers of participants using newer imaging techniques to detect cartilage damage.

Table 6.3 Commonly used hyaluronic acid products

Name	Number of injections	Molecular weight (kDa)
Hyalgan	5 at weekly intervals	615
		Low
Synvisc	3 at weekly intervals	6000
		High
Orthovisc	3 at weekly intervals	2000
		High
Hyalart	5 at weekly intervals	615
		Low
Arthrease	3 at weekly intervals	3000
		High
Durolane	1 injection	Polymer

Worldwide, there are a number of different HA products in clinical use, ranging from a single-dose injection to five injections at weekly intervals (Table 6.3).

Safety profile

There are no systemic adverse events associated with HA use. Local acute reactions at the injection site are not infrequent, up to 11% of injected knees in one report,[55] but are short-lived and merely require first-aid treatment. Acute aseptic arthritis, mimicking crystal arthritis, has been seen in association with 12 patients using Synvisc, a high molecular weight HA.[56] A retrospective study of 336 patients suggested that the incidence of local reactions is influenced by the injection technique: a medial approach and a partially flexed knee, 5.2%; a straight medial approach, 2.4%; and a straight lateral approach, 1.5%.[57]

What is the evidence?

Despite the number of clinical trials performed on intra-articular HA, debate remains about the degree of its effectiveness in patients with knee OA, predominantly due to the difficulties in assimilating evidence because of the differences in study design and the number of different HA preparations used. Two recent meta-analyses have examined the effects of intra-articular HA in knee OA. Both concluded that intra-articular HA was superior to an intra-articular placebo, and that the benefit of HA appeared to be greater in the smaller, less well-designed studies. The benefit was also less in studies that allowed paracetamol as escape analgesia, and possibly in those with more severe radiographic disease. There was some evidence that higher molecular weight HA resulted in greater pain relief than lower molecular weight HA. The meta-analyses disagreed on whether there was significant publication bias.[58,59]

The EULAR recommendations state that HAs have symptomatic effects in terms of both pain reduction and improvement in function.[4] One study investigated intra-articular corticosteroid versus intra-articular HA in 100 subjects. No differences between the treatment groups were found at the 6-month follow-up with respect to pain relief or function. Of more interest is that women demonstrated significantly less response to treatment than men, for both treatments and across all outcome measures.[60] Studies addressing possible predictors of response are few. Patients over 60 years with functional impairment, as documented by the Lequesne index, had greater efficacy with HA in one study.[61] A retrospective study found that the response to HA was statistically influenced by the structural severity of knee OA; those with less severe disease did better, and those with an effusion at baseline did worse.[57] It is noteworthy that the majority of trials investigating intra-articular HA exclude severe OA.

Summary

There is evidence to support the efficacy of HA in the management of OA, in terms of both pain reduction and functional improvement. However, although pain relief may be obtained for several months, rather than several weeks as with steroids, this benefit may be offset by its slower onset of action and by the requirement of a course of three to five injections at weekly intervals, with the logistical and cost issues that that entails. There is minimal evidence for a role in disease modification.

GLUCOSAMINE SULPHATE

Background

In much of Europe, glucosamine sulphate is a prescription drug, but in the US and the UK it remains an over-the-counter health supplement. Glucosamine

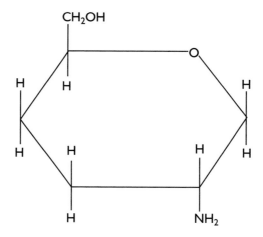

Figure 6.4 Chemical structure of glucosamine

sulphate and glucosamine hydrochloride have been subjected to clinical trials; most being conducted with glucosamine sulphate. It is thought that the sulphate moiety attached to glucosamine may confer some of the clinical effects observed.[62] Glucosamine has been suggested to have both a symptomatic effect on relieving pain and also a structure-modifying effect in OA.

Glucosamine consists of an amino acid group attached to glucose (Figure 6.4), and is a major constituent of various tissues within the joint, including cartilage. It has been reported to have both anti-inflammatory effects in animal models and direct effects on chondrocytes in human models. Glucosamine dose-dependently inhibits the pro-inflammatory cytokine interleukin-1;[63] such molecules reduce proteoglycan synthesis and therefore inhibit cartilage repair. Adding glucosamine to chondrocyte cultures increases proteoglycan synthesis. Glucosamine sulphate has also been shown to stimulate mRNA and protein levels of aggrecan core protein, and inhibit the production and enzymic activity of matrix-degrading matrix metalloproteinase-3 in chondrocytes, thereby preventing articular cartilage loss.[64] These mechanisms may explain some of the beneficial clinical effects seen.

A recent study suggests that degeneration of cartilage may be triggered by metabolic disorders of glucose balance, and that OA occurs coincident with metabolic disease and diabetes mellitus. The authors present a novel hypothesis about the role of glucose transport and metabolism in cartilage pathology, and speculate that supplementation with sugar-based compounds may benefit patients with OA.[65]

Safety profile

Glucosamine has been found to be a safe product, with a side-effect profile similar to that of placebo in placebo-controlled trials. Of nearly 1000 patients randomized to glucosamine in RCTs, only 14 withdrew due to toxicity.[66]

Due to its chemical structure, there has been concern that glucosamine may raise patients' plasma glucose levels and, therefore, theoretically potentiate the onset of insulin resistance or diabetes mellitus and make pre-existing disease worse. Two studies have examined the effects of intravenous glucosamine on healthy subjects, finding no effect on insulin sensitivity or plasma glucose levels.[67,68] A further study in patients with type II diabetes mellitus demonstrated that oral glucosamine hydrochloride 1500 mg daily plus chondroitin sulphate (CS) 1200 mg daily did not alter glycosylated haemoglobin levels, and suggested that glucosamine may be a safe alternative to other medications in patients with diabetes and OA.[69]

What is the evidence?

The symptomatic effects of glucosamine on OA have been studied since 1969. Most studies have found a beneficial effect, particularly in mild to moderate OA, although negative studies have been published.[70] A number of systematic reviews and meta-analyses have now been performed to collate these results. A Cochrane review[66] identified 16 RCTs, combining single-blind, double-blind, placebo and comparator studies; the ES for pain reduction, comparing glucosamine with placebo, was 1.4, representing a clinically significant ES; for function, the pooled SMD compared with placebo was 0.63. In those studies comparing glucosamine with NSAIDs (ibuprofen), the pooled SMD for pain reduction was 0.86, suggesting that glucosamine is an alternative to NSAID treatment; the NSAID group responded more quickly to treatment, although at the 8-week follow-up, the glucosamine group did significantly better. In all but one study, glucosamine sulphate was investigated. Of interest, in the study investigating glucosamine hydrochloride, no effect was found for glucosamine over placebo.[71]

A more recent meta-analysis included placebo-controlled studies of glucosamine sulphate and CS, pooling data for 1775 subjects.[72] The common ES for pain reduction was modest at 0.49, with no differences between glucosamine and chondroitin. In an earlier meta-analysis,[73] including fewer studies, there was a difference in ES between glucosamine and chondroitin (for glucosamine: small trials 0.5 and large trials 0.4; for chondroitin: small trials 1.7 and large trials 0.8). This meta-analysis, as with others,[73] has shown that there is undoubtedly a degree of publication bias, and therefore symptomatic effects may be mildly exaggerated. The minimal time reported for the onset of significant pain reduction was 2 weeks, but was generally in the region of 3 months. The authors also examined the potential disease-modifying role of glucosamine, finding a highly significant effect on joint-space narrowing of glucosamine 1500 mg daily, compared with placebo ($p < 0.001$), taken from two studies;[74,75] the global ES for this structure-modifying effect was 0.41. A sub-analysis from one of these studies suggests that subjects with less severe radiographic knee OA will experience more disease progression and may be more responsive to disease-modifying drugs.[76]

Summary

Glucosamine sulphate appears to have a mild–moderate effect on pain and may be an alternative or additional treatment for OA. The onset of action is slower than that seen with paracetamol or NSAIDs, and may be up to 3 months. Initial concerns about toxicity in patients with diabetes or insulin resistance may be unfounded. Two studies have demonstrated retardation in the progression of knee OA, suggesting it may also have a role in disease modification.

CHONDROITIN SULPHATE

Background

Chondroitin-4 and -6 sulphate are the most commonly found glycos-aminoglycans in cartilage. Due to its large molecular size, only 10–15% of CS is absorbed in the GI tract. It is manufactured from shark and bovine cartilage; careful selection of cattle is necessary to avoid herds contaminated with bovine spongiform encephalopathy.

Animal models have demonstrated cartilage protection by both oral and intravenous chondroitin supplementation. It has been postulated that CS, like glucosamine sulphate, has both a symptomatic and disease-modifying effect in patients with OA. The studies that have been conducted appear to have more consistently positive findings than those with glucosamine, although varying drug doses have been used.

Safety profile

No serious side-effects have been reported in the published trials.

What is the evidence?

A meta-analysis evaluated nine placebo-controlled trials; all reported a significant benefit with chondroitin, with a pooled ES from the better-quality trials of 0.8, which is considered large.[14] The efficacy of CS was compared with that of diclofenac; a more prompt reduction of clinical symptoms was seen with diclofenac, but these returned after treatment was stopped. CS had a slower onset of action, but this was maintained for up to 3 months after treatment was stopped.[77] Uebelhart and colleagues have investigated this apparently prolonged effect in a 12-month study of placebo compared with two intermittent 3-month treatment episodes of CS 800 mg.[78] They showed a significant symptomatic effect of CS, as well as an inhibitory effect of CS on radiological progression, suggesting a disease-modifying effect. Disease modification has also been suggested in pilot studies of hand OA,[79] in which those taking CS had less radiological progression and less erosive disease, compared with placebo, although CS did not appear to prevent OA from developing.

Patients in the community often take a combination of CS and glucosamine. Only one study, combining CS, glucosamine hydrochloride and manganese ascorbate, has addressed this;[80] patients with mild to moderate OA had a significant benefit, but those with severe disease showed a response similar to that with placebo.

Summary

CS appears to be safe and efficacious. There may be a disease-modifying effect but this requires further research. The evidence available suggests that CS is useful in patients with mild to moderate OA, and that it has a sustained effect, even after treatment is discontinued.

CONCLUSIONS

The drugs outlined all have some efficacy in relieving pain from OA, some more than others. Unfortunately, it is the norm for treatments to be investigated as monotherapy, when most would advocate a management plan incorporating both non-pharmacological and combination pharmacological therapy in a graded approach. Due to the heterogeneity of patients with OA, each patient and their disease needs to be catered for individually, with careful thought for the potential adverse effects of treatment weighed against the benefits in terms of improving pain and function and enabling the patient to maintain the normal activities of daily living.

*Note added in proof

As this book went to press, rofecoxib was withdrawn due to an increase in cardiovascular endpoints. Other COX-II inhibitors and some conventional NSAIDs are also being reappraised in light of potential adverse cardiovascular risk.

References

1. Schwarzer R 2004; Meta-analysis programs version 5.0 Berlin, Germany: Ralf Schwarzer Computer Programs for Meta-Analysis, 2000. (www.fuberlin.de/-gesund/meta_e.htm)

2. Mering von J. Beiträge zur Kenntniss der Antipyretica. Ther Monatshefte 1893; 7: 578

3. Kaufman DW, Kelly JP, Anderson TE, Mitchell AA. A comprehensive ongoing population-based survey of medication use in the United States: the adult population. Pharmacoepidemiol Drug Saf 2000; 9: S60

4. Jordan KM, Arden N, Doherty M, et al. EULAR Recommendations 2003: an evidence based approach to the management of knee osteoarthritis: report of a Task Force of the Standing Committee for International Clinical Studies Including Therapeutic Trials (ESCISIT). Ann Rheum Dis 2003; 62: 1145–55

5. American College of Rheumatology Subcommittee on Osteoarthritis Guidelines. Recommendations for the medical management of osteoarthritis of the hip and knee. Arthritis Rheum 2000; 43: 1905–15

6. Rodriguez LAG, Hernandez-Diaz S. Relative risk of upper gastrointestinal complications among users of acetaminophen and nonsteroidal anti-inflammatory drugs. Epidemiology 2001; 12: 570–6

7. Rahme E, Pettitt D, LeLorier J. Determinants and sequelae associated with utilisation of acetaminophen versus traditional nonsteroidal antiinflammatory drugs in an elderly population. Arthritis Rheum 2002; 46: 3046–54

8. Schneitman-McIntyre O, Farnen TA, Gordon N, et al. Medication misadventures resulting in emergency department visits at HMO Medical Centre. Am J Health Syst Pharm 1996; 53: 1422

9. Benson GD. Acetaminophen in chronic liver disease. Clin Pharmacol Ther 1983; 33: 95–101

10. Amadio P, Cummings DM. Evaluation of acetaminophen in the management of osteoarthritis of the knee. Curr Ther Res 1983; 34: 59–66

11. Bradley JD, Brandt KD, Katz BP, et al. Treatment of knee osteoarthritis: relationship of clinical features of joint inflammation to the response to a nonsteroidal antiinflammatory drug or pure analgesic. J Rheumatol 1992; 19: 1950–4

12. Bradley JD, Katz BP, Brandt KD. Severity of knee pain does not predict a better response to an antiinflammatory dose of ibuprofen than to analgesic therapy in patients with osteoarthritis. J Rheumatol 2001; 28: 1073–6

13. Williams HJ, Ward JR, Egger MJ, et al. Comparison of naproxen and acetaminophen in a two year study of treatment of osteoarthritis of the knee. Arthritis Rheum 1993; 36: 1196–206

14. Pincus T, Koch GG, Sokka T, et al. A randomized, double-blind, crossover clinical trial of diclofenac plus misoprostol versus acetaminophen in patients with osteoarthritis of the hip or knee. Arthritis Rheum 2001; 44: 1587–98

15. Geba GP, Weaver AL, Polis AB, et al. Efficacy of rofecoxib, celecoxib, and acetaminophen in osteoarthritis of the knee: a randomized trial. J Am Med Assoc 2002; 287: 64–71

16. Case JP, Baliunas AJ, Block JA. Lack of efficacy of acetaminophen in treating symptomatic knee osteoarthritis: a randomised, double blind, placebo-controlled comparison trial with diclofenac. Arch Intern Med 2003; 163: 169–78

17. Pincus T, Swearingen C, Cummins P, Callahan LF. Preference for nonsteroidal antiinflammatory drugs versus acetaminophen and concomitant use of both types of drugs in patients with osteoarthritis. J Rheumatol 2000; 27: 1020–7

18. Towheed TE, Judd M, Hochberg MC, Wells G. Acetaminophen for osteoarthritis. Cochrane Database Syst Rev 2003: CD004257

19. Jones R. Nonsteroidal anti-inflammatory drug prescribing: past, present, and future. Am J Med 2001; 110: 4S–7S

20. Brun J, Jones R. Nonsteroidal anti-inflammatory drug-associated dyspepsia: the scale of the problem. Am J Med 2001; 110: 12S–13S

21. Silverstein FE, Faich G, Goldstein JL, et al. Gastrointestinal toxicity with celecoxib vs nonsteroidal anti-inflammatory drugs for osteoarthritis and rheumatoid arthritis. J Am Med Assoc 2000; 284: 1247–55

22. Goldstein JL, Silverstein FE, Agrawal N, et al. Reduced risk of upper gastrointestinal ulcer complications with celecoxib, a novel COX-2 inhibitor. Am J Gastroenterol 2000; 95: 1681–90

23. Goldstein JL, Correa P, Zhao WW, et al. Reduced incidence of gastrointestinal ulcers with celecoxib, a novel cyclooxygenase-2 inhibitor, compared to naproxen in patients with arthritis. Am J Gastroenterol 2004; 96: 1019–27

24. Goldstein JL, Zhao SZ, Burke TA, et al. Incidence of outpatient physician claims for upper gastrointestinal symptoms among new users of celecoxib, ibuprofen and naproxen in an insured population in the United States. Am J Gastroenterol 2003; 98: 2627–34

25. Mamdani M, Juurlink DN, Lee DS, et al. Cyclo-oxygenase-2 inhibitors versus non-selective non-steroidal anti-inflammatory drugs and congestive heart failure outcomes in elderly patients: a population based cohort study. Lancet 2004; 363: 1751–6

26. Wolfe F, Zhao S, Pettitt D. Blood pressure destabilization and edema among 8538 users of celecoxib, rofecoxib, and nonselective nonsteroidal antiinflammatory drugs (NSAID) and nonusers of NSAID receiving ordinary clinical care. J Rheumatol 2004; 31: 1143–51

27. Howard PA, Delafontaine P. Nonsteroidal anti-inflammatory drugs and cardiovascular risk. J Am Coll Cardiol 2004; 43: 519–25

28. Towheed TE, Shea B, Wells G, Hochberg M. Analgesia and non-aspirin, non-steroidal anti-inflammatory drugs for osteoarthritis of the hip. Cochrane Library 2003; Issue 2 (Oxford: Update Software)

29. Watson MC, Brookes ST, Kirwan JR, Faulkner A. Non-aspirin, non-steroidal anti-inflammatory drugs for osteoarthritis of the knee. Cochrane Database Syst Rev 2000: CD000142

30. Day R, Morrison B, Luza A, et al. A randomized trial of the efficacy and tolerability of the COX-2 inhibitor rofecoxib vs ibuprofen in patients with osteoarthritis. Rofecoxib/Ibuprofen Comparator Study Group. Arch Intern Med 2000; 160: 1781–7

31. Saag K, van-der-Heijde D, Fisher C, et al. Rofecoxib, a new cyclooxygenase 2 inhibitor, shows sustained efficacy, comparable with other nonsteroidal anti-inflammatory drugs: a 6-week and a 1-year trial in patients with osteoarthritis. Osteoarthritis Studies Group. Arch Fam Med 2000; 9: 1124–34

32. Cannon GW, Caldwell JR, Holt P, et al. Rofecoxib, a specific inhibitor of cyclooxygenase 2, with clinical efficacy comparable with that of diclofenac sodium: results of a one-year, randomized, clinical trial in patients with osteoarthritis of the knee and hip. Rofecoxib Phase III Protocol 035 Study Group. Arthritis Rheum 2000; 43: 978–87

33. Bensen WG, Fiechtner JJ, McMillen JI, et al. Treatment of osteoarthritis with celecoxib, a cyclooxygenase-2 inhibitor: a randomized controlled trial. Mayo Clin Proc 1999; 74: 1095–105

34. McKenna F, Borenstein D, Wendt H, et al. Celecoxib versus diclofenac in the management of osteoarthritis of the knee. Scand J Rheumatol 2001; 30: 11–18

35. Huskisson EC, Macciocchi A, Rahlfs VW, et al. Nimesulide versus diclofenac in the treatment of osteoarthritis of the hip or knee: an active controlled equivalence study. Curr Ther Res 1999; 60: 253–65

36. Scott DL, Berry H, Capell H, et al. The long-term effects of non-steroidal anti-inflammatory drugs in osteoarthritis of the knee: a randomized placebo-controlled trial. Rheumatology (Oxford) 2000; 39: 1095–101

37. Kriegel W, Korff KJ, Ehrlich JC, et al. Double-blind study comparing the long-term efficacy of the COX-2 inhibitor nimesulide and naproxen in patients with osteoarthritis. Int J Clin Pract 2001; 55: 510–14

38. Dickson DJ. A double blind evaluation of topical piroxicam gel with oral ibuprofen in osteoarthritis of the knee. Curr Ther Res 1991; 49: 199–207

39. Evans JM, McMahon AD, McGilchrist MM, et al. Topical non-steroidal anti-inflammatory drugs and admission to hospital for upper gastrointestinal bleeding and perforation: a record linkage case control study. Br Med J 1995; 311: 22–6

40. Moore RA, Tramer MR, Carroll D, et al. Quantitative systematic review of topically applied non-steroidal anti-inflammatory drugs. Br Med J 1998; 316: 333–8

41. Ottillinger B, Gomor B, Michel BA, et al. Efficacy and safety of eltenac gel in the treatment of knee osteoarthritis. Osteoarthritis Cartilage 2001; 9: 273–80

42. Grace D, Rogers J, Skeith K, Anderson K. Topical diclofenac versus placebo: a double blind, randomized clinical trial in patients with osteoarthritis of the knee. J Rheumatol 1999; 26: 2659–63

43. van-Haselen RA, Fisher PA. A randomized controlled trial comparing topical piroxicam gel with a homeopathic gel in osteoarthritis of the knee. Rheumatology (Oxford) 2000; 39: 714–19

44. Deal CL, Schnitzer TJ, Lipstein IE, et al. Treatment of arthritis with topical capsaicin: a double-blind trial. Clin Ther 1991; 13: 383–95

45. McCarthy GM, McCarty DJ. Effect of topical capsaicin in the therapy of painful osteoarthritis of the hands. J Rheumatol 1992; 19: 604–7

46. McCleane G. The analgesic efficacy of topical capsaicin is enhanced by glyceryl trinitrate in painful osteoarthritis: a randomized, double blind, placebo controlled study. Eur J Pain 2000; 4: 355–60

47. Chakravarty K, Pharaoh PDP, Scott DGI. A randomised controlled study of post injection rest following intra-articular steroid therapy for knee synovitis. Br J Rheumatol 1994; 33: 464–8

48. Raynauld JP, Buckland-Wright C, Ward R, et al. Safety and efficacy of long-term intraarticular steroid injections in osteoarthritis of the knee: a randomized, double-blind, placebo-controlled trial. Arthritis Rheum 2003; 48: 370–7

49. Hollander JL. Intrasynovial corticosteroid therapy in arthritis. Md State Med J 1970; 19: 62–6

50. Arroll B, Goodyear-Smith F. Corticosteroid injections for osteoarthritis of the knee: meta-analysis. Br Med J 2004; 328: 869

51. Gaffney VK, Ledingham J, Perry JD. Intra-articular triamcinalone hexacetonide in knee osteoarthritis: factors influencing the clinical response. Ann Rheum Dis 1995; 54: 379–81

52. Jones A, Doherty M. Intra-articular corticosteroids are effective in osteoarthritis but there are no clinical predictors of response. Ann Rheum Dis 1996; 55: 829–32

53. Balazs EA. Hyaluronic acid and matrix implantation. Arlington (MA): Biotrix Inc, 1971

54. Dahl LB, Dahl IMS, Engstrom-Laurent A, Granath K. Concentration and molecular weight of sodium hyaluronate in synovial fluid from patients with rheumatoid arthritis and other arthropathies. Ann Rheum Dis 1985; 44: 817–22

55. Puttick MPE, Wade JP, Chalmers A, et al. Acute local reactions after intra articular Hylan for osteoarthritis of the knee. J Rheumatol 1995; 22: 1311–14

56. Bernardeau C, Bucki B, Liote F. Acute arthritis after intra-articular hyaluronate injection: onset of effusions without crystal. Ann Rheum Dis 2001; 60: 518–20

57. Lussier A, Cividino AA, McFarlane CA, et al. Viscosupplementation with hylan for the treatment of osteoarthritis: findings from clinical practice in Canada. J Rheumatol 1996; 23: 1579–85

58. Lo GH, La Valley M, McAlindon T, Felson DT. Intra-articular hyaluronic acid in treatment of knee osteoarthritis: a meta-analysis. J Am Med Assoc 2003; 290: 3115–21

59. Wang CT, Lin J, Chang CJ, et al. Therapeutic effects of hyaluronic acid on osteoarthritis of the knee. A meta-analysis of randomized controlled trials. J Bone Joint Surg Am 2004; 86: 538–45

60. Leopold SS, Redd BB, Warmw WJ, et al. Corticosteroid compared with hyaluronic acid injections for treatment of osteoarthritis of the knee. A prospective, randomized controlled trial. J Bone Joint Surg Am 2003; 85: 1197–203

61. Lohmander LS, Dalen N, Englund G. Intra-articular hyaluronan injections in the treatment of osteoarthritis of the knee: a randomised, double blind, placebo-controlled multicentre trial. Ann Rheum Dis 1996; 55: 424–31

62. Hoffer LJ, Kaplan LN, Hamadeh MJ, et al. Sulfate could mediate the therapeutic effect of glucosamine sulfate. Metabolism 2001; 50: 767–70

63. Gouze JN, Bordji K, Gulberti S. Interleukin-1beta down-regulates the expression of glucuronosyltransferase I, a key enzyme priming glycosaminoglycan biosynthesis: influence of glucosamine on interleukin-1beta-mediated effects in rat chondrocytes. Arthritis Rheum 2001; 44: 351–60

64. Dodge GR, Jimenez SA. Glucosamine sulfate modulates the levels of aggrecan and matrix metalloproteinase 3 synthesized by cultured human osteoarthritis articular chondrocytes. Osteoarthritis Cartilage 2003; 11: 424–32

65. Mobasheri A, Vannucci SJ, Bondy CA, et al. Glucose transport and metabolism in chondrocytes: a key to understanding chondrogenesis, skeletal development and cartilage degradation in osteoarthritis. Histol Histopathol 2002; 17: 1239–67

66. Towheed TE, Anastassiades TP, Shea B, et al. Glucosamine therapy for treating osteoarthritis. Cochrane Database Syst Rev 2001: CD002946

67. Pouwels M, Jacobs J, Span P, et al. Short-term glucosamine infusion does not affect insulin sensitivity in humans. J Clin Endocrinol Metab 2001; 86: 2099–103

68. Monauni T, Zenti M, Croft P, et al. Effects of glucosamine infusion on insulin secretion and insulin action in humans. Diabetes 2000; 49: 926–35

69. Scroggie DA, Albright A, Harris MD. The effect of glucosamine-chondroitin supplementation on glycosylated hemoglobin levels in patients with type 2 diabetes. Arch Intern Med 2003; 163: 1587–90

70. Hughes R, Carr A. A randomized, double-blind, placebo-controlled trial of glucosamine sulphate as an analgesic in osteoarthritis of the knee. Rheumatology (Oxford) 2002; 41: 279–84

71. Houpt JB, McMillan R, Wein C, Paget-Dellio SD. Effect of glucosamine hydrochloride in the treatment of pain of osteoarthritis of the knee. J Rheumatol 1999; 26: 2423–30

72. Richy F, Bruyere O, Ethgen O, et al. Structural and symptomatic efficacy of glucosamine and chondroitin in knee osteoarthritis. Arch Intern Med 2003; 163: 1514–22

73. McAlindon TE, LaValley MP, Gulin JP, Felson DT. Glucosamine and chondroitin for treatment of osteoarthritis: a systematic quality assessment and meta-analysis. J Am Med Assoc 2000; 283: 1469–75

74. Pavelka K, Gatterova J, Olejarova M, et al. Glucosamine sulfate use and delay of progression of knee osteoarthritis: a 3-year, randomized, placebo-controlled, double-blind study. Arch Intern Med 2002; 162: 2113–23

75. Reginster JY, Deroisy R, Rovati LC, et al. Long-term effects of glucosamine sulphate on osteoarthritis progression: a randomised, placebo-controlled clinical trial. Lancet 2001; 357: 251–6

76. Bruyere O, Honore A, Ethgen O, et al. Correlation between radiographic severity of knee osteoarthritis and future disease progression. Results from a 3-year prospective, placebo-controlled study evaluating the effect of glucosamine sulfate. Osteoarthritis Cartilage 2003; 11: 1–5

77. Morreale P, Manopulo R, Galati M, et al. Comparison of the antiinflammatory efficacy of chondroitin sulphate and diclofenac sodium in patients with knee osteoarthritis. J Rheumatol 1996; 23: 1385–91

78. Uebelhart D, Malaise M, Marcolongo R, et al. Intermittent treatment of knee osteoarthritis with oral chondroitin sulfate: a one-year, randomized, double-blind, multicenter study versus placebo. Osteoarthritis Cartilage 2004; 12: 269–76

79. Verbruggen G, Goemare S, Veys EM. Systems to assess the progression of finger joint osteoarthritis and the effects of disease modifying osteoarthritis drugs. Clin Rheumatol 2002; 21: 231–43

80. Das AJ, Hammad TA. Efficacy of a combination of FCHG49 glucosamine hydrochloride, TRH122 low molecular weight sodium chondroitin sulfate and manganese ascorbate in the management of knee osteoarthritis. Osteoarthritis Cartilage 2000; 8: 343–50

7

Surgical treatment of osteoarthritis

L Stefan Lohmander, Sören Toksvig-Larsen

KEY POINTS

- Surgical treatment options for the osteoarthritic joint include debridement and lavage; penetration of the subchondral bone; joint resection; transplantation of soft tissue, osteochondral grafts or chondrocytes, or implantation of artificial matrices; osteotomy; and endoprosthetic joint replacement.

- Endoprosthetic joint replacement of the hip and knee is a common, safe and successful procedure. It is based on Charnley's original design in which a metal head articulates against a polyethylene cup. These parts are often fixed to bone using an acrylic polymer.

- Subsequent improvements in the design and technique of joint replacement have greatly reduced the failure rate, but revision surgery is sometimes needed for loosening, wear or infection.

- Several of the methods for preservation or regeneration of a damaged joint surface have led to generation of new joint tissue and relief of symptoms. However, patient series are small, results appear to deteriorate with time, and the specific indications for individual methods remain uncertain.

- None of the techniques for joint preservation, with the exception, perhaps, of osteotomy, has shown a durable effect in osteoarthritis. Randomized controlled trials that compare the benefits and risks of these different techniques with the natural history of the disease are lacking.

INTRODUCTION

Osteoarthritis (OA) is associated with a slow and gradual deterioration of the joint. The main symptoms are joint pain, stiffness and limited mobility, which may lead to impairment and handicap. OA sometimes leads to the destruction of the joint and the need for an operation to replace the joint. However, for most patients with OA, surgical treatment never becomes necessary, and their problems can be treated satisfactorily by the management options described elsewhere in this book (Figure 7.1).

OA is not a single disease, but should rather be seen as a common final stage – joint failure – where the initial process can be triggered by many different causes. When the disease is far advanced, a routine X-ray examination will show reduced joint space and osteophytes. These changes to the structure of the joint are caused by destruction of the articular cartilage and growth of bone at the margins of the joints. Today, there is no treatment that can, with certainty, stop the progress of the osteoarthritic disease, but there is a series of treatments that can reduce the pain and help maintain or improve function. This chapter describes the surgical options for treating OA, most often reserved for the more severe stages of the disease.

Joint replacement dominates the surgical options for the treatment of osteoarthritic joints, but procedures that aim to preserve or restore articular cartilage, instead of replacing it with synthetic materials, provide alternatives.

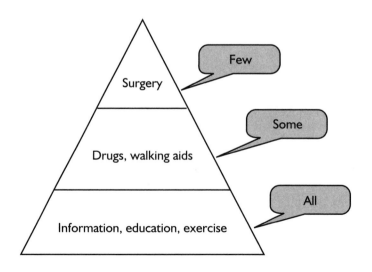

Figure 7.1 Principles of the management of osteoarthritis

These procedures can, for some younger patients with OA and localized loss or early articular cartilage damage, maintain or restore joint structure; this may allow a high level of physical activity, and delay or even eliminate the need for joint replacement.

Endoprosthetic joint replacement is of proven value in the treatment of OA of the hip, knee, shoulder and some other joints. The introduction of joint replacement has transformed the lives of OA patients with severe pain and functional impairment.

TREATMENTS THAT ATTEMPT TO PROTECT OR RESTORE ARTICULAR CARTILAGE

Joint debridement and lavage

Joint debridement includes joint irrigation, resection of cartilage flaps and removal of loose meniscal fragments,[1,2] and may include shaving of degenerated meniscal and articular cartilage surfaces.[3–5] Removal of osteochondral and meniscal fragments that cause mechanical disturbances of joint function has been reported to improve function and decrease symptoms.[6,7] The potential benefits of other debridement procedures are less clear.

Despite widespread use, shaving or debriding fibrillated articular cartilage and menisci remains controversial.[8,9] A recent double-blinded, randomized controlled trial involving arthroscopic debridement, arthroscopic lavage and arthroscopic surgery for knee OA compared outcome after 2 years with sham surgery.[10] At no time-point in this trial did either of the intervention groups report less pain or better function than the placebo group treated with sham surgery only. The outcome of this important trial shows that the symptomatic improvement sometimes observed after these procedures probably results from a placebo effect. This result emphasizes the significant role of the placebo effect in the surgical treatment of painful joints, and underlines the need for similar randomized controlled studies of other related treatments described in this chapter.

Penetration of subchondral bone

Penetration of subchondral bone may be used to stimulate the formation of a new articular surface by disrupting subchondral blood vessels, leading to the formation of a fibrin clot over the bone surface. Undifferentiated mesenchymal cells can migrate into the clot, proliferate and differentiate into cells with features of chondrocytes, which may form a fibrocartilage-like repair tissue.[11] It is unclear which method of penetrating subchondral bone produces the best new articular surface. In many individuals, the treatment results in the formation of tissue that varies in composition, from dense fibrous tissue to hyaline cartilage-like tissue. However, no studies have documented a relationship between the extent and type of repair tissue and the symptomatic or functional results. Despite the evidence that penetration of subchondral bone stimulates the formation of fibrocartilaginous repair tissue, and reports of symptomatic improvement in several series of patients, the long-term value remains uncertain. Short periods of follow-up, lack of well-defined outcome evaluations, lack of randomized controlled trials and the possibility for a significant placebo effect make it very difficult to define the indications in OA for these procedures.[10]

Resection arthroplasty

Resection of an osteoarthritic joint surface followed by joint motion results in the formation of connective tissue and fibrocartilage over the surfaces of the resected bone.[12] Resection arthroplasty is most successful in joints that do not require a high degree of stability, and where shortening due to resection of bone does not prevent function. One of the most commonly performed resection arthroplasties, the Keller arthroplasty (performed to treat hallux rigidus and OA of the first metatarsophalangeal joint), consists of resecting damaged articular cartilage along with the proximal portion of the proximal phalanx of the great toe. Following surgery, patients gradually begin active motion of the joint and often develop a satisfactory range of motion with minimal discomfort.

Soft tissue and cartilage grafts

Treatment of osteoarthritic joints by soft-tissue grafts involves interposing fascia, muscle, tendon, periosteum or perichondrium between debrided or resected articular surfaces. Soft-tissue interposition arthroplasties have been used most frequently to treat osteoarthritic joints of the upper extremities; in particular, tendon or fascia arthroplasty treatment of OA of the thumb carpometacarpal joint.[13] This procedure has often been found to provide relief of symptoms and to retain some joint motion.

Compared with soft-tissue grafts, cartilage or meniscal grafts have the advantage of more closely resembling the structure and composition of articular cartilage, and have the potential for transplantation of viable chondrocytes. Osteochondral allografts have been used to replace damaged segments of articular surfaces. More recent developments in this area include the use of autogenous osteochondral grafts taken from non-load-bearing areas of the knee joint, and transferred to areas of cartilage damage in the same knee, so-called mosaicplasty.[14] However, the value of these techniques has not been proven in the osteoarthritic joint.

Treatment with cells and growth factors

The limited ability of host cells to restore articular surfaces has led investigators to seek methods of transplanting cells that can form cartilage into chondral and osteochondral defects. Thus, autologous chondrocyte transplants have been used for the treatment of localized cartilage defects.[15,16] Results indicate that chondrocyte transplantation combined with a periosteal graft can, in some cases, promote restoration of an articular surface in humans. Further work and larger patient series are needed to assess if it improves joint function and delays or prevents future OA, and if this approach will be beneficial in osteoarthritic joints.

No blinded, controlled and randomized trials have yet been published that compare the patient-relevant outcomes of different methods of regeneration or repair of the injured joint cartilage with the natural history. The clinical series published have contained limited numbers of patients with variable forms and locations of joint damage, and the outcome measures used to report the results have too rarely been standardized, validated or patient-relevant.[17] Therefore, it may be that the results reported are associated with significant patient, examiner and publishing bias. The specific indications for, and the value of, these methods remain to be defined, in particular for the osteoarthritic joint.

Osteotomies

Treatment of an osteoarthritic joint with an osteotomy consists of cutting the bone adjacent to the involved joint and then stabilizing the cut bone surfaces in a new position, thereby changing the alignment and the resulting load of the joint surfaces. Osteotomies are planned to decrease loads on the most severely damaged regions of the joint surface, and correct joint malalignment that may be contributing to symptoms (Figure 7.2). Osteotomies of the hip and knee may decrease symptoms and stimulate the formation of a new articular surface. However, the mechanisms of symptomatic improvement and formation of new articular surfaces remain poorly understood. The decreased pain may result from reduced stresses on regions of the articular surface with the most advanced cartilage degeneration, reduced intraosseous pressure or the formation of a new articular surface. Reports of the treatment of knee OA with osteotomies describe an increased radiographic joint space, accompanied by decreased subchondral sclerosis and, in some people, formation of a new fibrocartilage articular surface.[18–20] However, no correlation has been found between histological score, radiographic appearance, post-operative varus–valgus angle or clinical results.

The overall clinical results of hip and knee osteotomies vary more than those of joint replacement, and our understanding is limited of the relationships between the degree of alteration of joint loading, type of osteotomy, quality and extent of articular surface repair, radiographic changes and clinical outcome.[21–23] Variables that appear adversely to affect the results of a knee osteotomy include advanced patient age, obesity, severe joint degeneration, joint instability, limited joint motion, operative overcorrection or undercorrection, and post-operative loss of correction.[21–26] Several studies report, however, that the results of osteotomies may be improved through better technique and patient selection, and may compare favourably with unicompartmental arthroplasty in young and physically active patients, although this remains to be proven in randomized controlled trials.[27]

Disadvantages of the commonly used 'bone wedge removal' osteotomies are loss of correction during healing, and a long period of fixation in a cast during healing of the osteotomy. The recently introduced method of callus distraction (hemicallotasis) osteotomy attempts to improve on these disadvantages. In this technique, pins are drilled into the bone on each side of a single-cut osteotomy, and an external frame attached (Figure 7.3). The frame is then slowly adjusted by the patient over the course of several weeks to months. During this time, the resulting defect is filled by callus and bone. When the correct angular correction is reached, the frame is locked in place until the defect is completely healed. The patient is allowed full weight-bearing during the treatment. Early results are encouraging, but longer follow-up of large patient series is needed to confirm the value of this technique.[28]

Tibial osteotomy is best suited for patients under 60 years of age with a stable knee and (preferably) OA located in the medial compartment, and with high

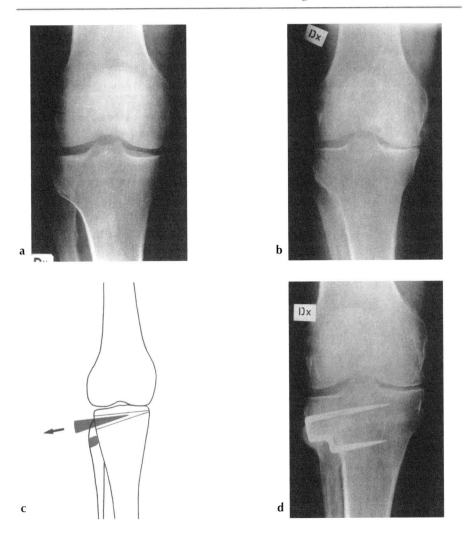

Figure 7.2 (a) X-ray film (standing anteroposterior) of right knee of a 44-year-old male. Medial meniscectomy was performed at age 34 years. The patient now has intermittent knee pain when walking, and some functional limitations. No radiological signs of osteoarthritis (OA), but borderline narrowing of medial joint space. (b) X-ray film of the same patient 13 years later (age 57 years). The patient now complains of persistent knee pain on walking, resting pain and sometimes night pain, with significant functional limitations. The radiograph shows medial osteophytes, loss of medial joint space. OA clinically and radiologically. (c) High tibial osteotomy of right knee performed at age 57 years. Lateral bone wedge removed to decrease load in medial compartment. (d) X-ray film of same knee performed 2 years later, at age 59 years. Osteotomy healed. Apparent increase in medial joint space. Improved walking distance, significant decrease in pain. From *Osteoarthritis*, 2nd edn. Oxford University Press, 2003, with permission

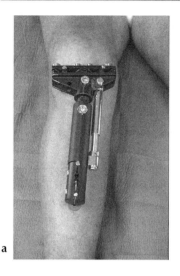
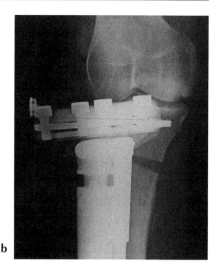

a   b

Figure 7.3 (a) and (b) Callus distraction osteotomy (hemicallotasis) of right knee, with external fixation applied. External fixator is gradually adjusted until planned correction with medial opening wedge is obtained. Osteotomy callus tissue is then allowed to heal and the fixator removed. Full weight-bearing and activity allowed during treatment

expectations of physical activity. If carried out on the right patient and with care, the result of an osteotomy is good and 'lasts' as long as a single-compartment, joint-replacement operation. Rehabilitation may be demanding, which is one reason for the upper age limit.

Conclusions

The efficacy of surgical treatments that attempt to preserve or restore articular cartilage has not been shown by prospective, randomized controlled studies, and the basic mechanisms by which they may relieve pain and improve function remain poorly understood.[17] Generally, these procedures produce less predictable results than joint replacement, and their efficacy, as measured by relief of symptoms and improved function, varies among joints, patients and procedures. Future surgical methods for preserving and restoring articular surfaces will need to begin with an analysis of the structural and functional abnormalities of the involved joint, and the patient's expectations for future joint use. The treatment plan will need to combine correction of joint malalignment and instability with methods to stimulate the regeneration of a functional joint cartilage.

ENDOPROSTHETIC JOINT REPLACEMENT

Referral for surgical treatment of OA

'Candidates for elective total hip replacement should have radiographic evidence of joint damage and moderate to severe persistent pain and/or disability that is not substantially relieved by an extended course of non-surgical management.' This summary recommendation was presented in 1994 at the National Institutes of Health as a conclusion of a consensus development conference on total hip replacement. While this recommendation still largely holds, it may not always be helpful in the evaluation of individual cases. With increasing experience and results, the age range of patients treated with total joint replacement is now being broadened to include more elderly patients with significant co-morbidities, as well as younger patients whose implants may be exposed to greater stresses over a longer time. Thus, with expanding use, the decisions may become less straightforward (Figure 7.4). As an aid to the setting of priorities in referrals and waiting lists, and in an attempt to move away from the simple 'can't sleep, can't work, can't walk' criterion for surgery, point systems have been presented and tested for priority setting for waiting lists and surgery (Figure 7.5).[29,30] However, a needs assessment for total joint replacement must also take into consideration other factors, such as willingness.[31,32]

Hip arthroplasty

The technique and design of the hip arthroplasty is based on the work of Charnley.[33] It relies on replacement of the femoral head and acetabulum with a metal femoral shaft and head articulating against a plastic acetabular cup (Figure 7.6). These components are fixed in the host bone by the use of a polymethyl metacrylate resin, giving a self-curing filler that bridges the gap between the stem of the hip prosthesis and the inside of the femoral shaft. Once cured, the substance is inert and fixes the components to the bone. Low friction and durability are achieved by a small femoral head diameter and an acetabular cup of high-density polyethylene. Charnley's low-friction arthroplasty is finalized with a set of orthopaedic instruments and strict surgical routines.

Hundreds of similar designs have subsequently been introduced on the market, some resulting in incremental improvements in outcome, and some of them major failures. The original design concept as developed by Charnley has proved challenging to improve upon significantly.

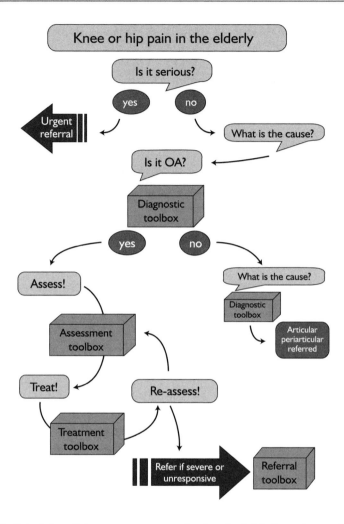

Figure 7.4 Principles of the management and referral of elderly patients with knee or hip pain. OA, osteoarthritis

The early years of hip arthroplasty were associated with high rates of deep infection, which were reduced significantly by the introduction of clean air operating enclosures, improved operating gowns, etc. Further reduction of the infection rate has been achieved with prophylactic antibiotics given during surgery or added to the bone cement for slow release locally.

Other technical developments have focused on the bone cement, attempting to increase the strength of the cement and its interface with the implant and the host bone. Mixing in a partial vacuum is now a common technique to decrease

Priority criteria for major joint replacement
(maximum points 100)

- PAIN 40
  - Severity 0–20, Duration 0–20

- FUNCTION 20
  - Walking difficulty 0–10
  - Other 0–10

- JOINT DAMAGE 20
  - Pain on passive movement 0–10
  - Other/X-ray 0–10

- OTHER 20
  - Other joints 0–10
  - Work, care giving, independence 0–10

Figure 7.5 Summary of priority criteria for major joint replacement. Further details are available in the publication by Hadorn and Holmes[29]

cement porosity and improve fatigue properties. However, mechanical loosening (not associated with e.g. deep infection) remains a major reason for arthroplasty re-operations (revision surgery). Therefore, much effort is being spent on 'biological' fixation methods, with direct bone-to-implant contact.

The most recent developments in solving the durable fixation of the acetabular cup is a solid metal shell with a smooth inner surface that makes full contact with the plastic cup liner. The metal shell is porous-coated on the outside to encourage ingrowth of host bone in the absence of bone cement. This type of acetabular implant may be as reliable as cemented acetabular cups.

Porous coating for biological fixation is also used in the femoral shaft.[34] The technique requires a large number of implant sizes to allow optimal filling of the medullary cavity of the femur for a stable fit (Figure 7.7). Initial stability is essential for bone ingrowth, and as little as 150 μm of micromotion will prevent it. The natural variability in the shape of the proximal femur makes it impossible to obtain more than isolated areas with good bone-to-implant contact. Early models of porous coating femoral prostheses for bone ingrowth have shown a higher rate of loosening than the traditional cemented designs. New and improved designs are being introduced, but proof of long-term advantages is still lacking.[35] In continued efforts to solve the problem of prosthesis loosening, bioactive coatings such as hydroxyapatite are now being tested to create a stronger bond between the implant and the host bone. As with any new hip arthroplasty design, long-term follow-up data are needed to evaluate properly the clinical and patient-relevant value of these new concepts.

With improvements in the durability of hip prostheses, implant wear in the articulation between the femoral head and the acetabular cup has increased as a concern. This has led to improvement in the surface quality of the femoral heads and the use of ceramic heads or metal-to-metal articulations (Figure 7.7). Modern metal-to-plastic implants have a wear rate of 0.1–0.2 mm per year.

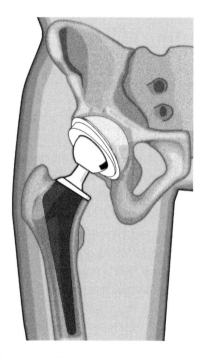

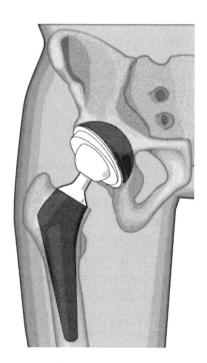

Figure 7.6 Cemented hip prosthesis with a smooth stem, a modular 28-mm head and a high-density polyethylene plastic cup, a design based on the low-friction arthroplasty of Charnley. From *Osteoarthritis*, 2nd edn. Oxford University Press, 2003, with permission

Figure 7.7 Cementless hip prosthesis in which the femoral stem and acetabular cup are covered with a porous surface to encourage bone ingrowth in order to give fixation against the cortical bone. The femoral head is ceramic for wear reduction. From *Osteoarthritis*, 2nd edn. Oxford University Press, 2003, with permission

Currently used hip prostheses and results

Sales statistics in Europe show that total hip arthroplasties are most often carried out with cemented femoral stems, while cemented and uncemented cups are equally common. In Scandinavia, a cemented total hip replacement with a cobalt-chromium-molybdenum or stainless steel femoral component articulating against a polyethylene acetabular cup is commonly used. Use of a cement-restricting plug, careful cleaning of the bone bed, and cement pressurization of vacuum-mixed cement with a gun is standard practice.[36] The cumulative revision rate for infection is reported to be 0.5% at 10 years with the use of ultraclean air filtration and antibiotic-containing bone cement. The overall 10-year revision rate for loosening is 6–7% for surgery performed in the 1990s; higher in men and in younger patients. Further differences are apparent when comparing the risk of revision between different diagnoses; surgery in connection with femoral neck fracture or rheumatoid arthritis has a higher risk than OA. The current cumulative 10-year risk for hip implant revision surgery due to loosening is 5% for patients with OA.[37] Modern cemented implants differ little in revision rate. However, the experience with uncemented implants, to date, has not encouraged their widespread, continued use. This conclusion is supported by the Norwegian Arthroplasty Register, in which uncemented implants had twice as high a risk of revision as the cemented implants, and even higher among younger patients.[38]

Following hip replacement, hip pain and function improve rapidly, but at least 1 year is needed to assess the full benefits of the intervention (Figure 7.8).[39,40] At 1 year after hip replacement, the quality of life of the patient is comparable to that of the age- and sex-matched general population.[37,39,40] However, individual outcome is variable and there is a need for improved criteria for pre-operative identification of 'non-responders'.[40]

Knee arthroplasty

Early clinical experience of knee arthroplasty was rewarding, with good mobility, stability and pain relief. However, the failure rate was higher than that with contemporary hip arthroplasties, due to loosening and deep infection. Continued developments have led to a decrease in implant size, guide instruments to ensure proper alignment of the leg, position of the implant and soft tissue balance, and improved fixation techniques.

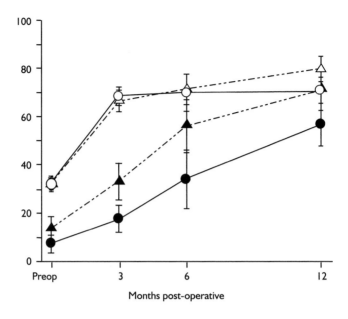

Figure 7.8 Change in the SF-36 sub-scales 'Role Function' and 'Bodily Pain' during 12 months following total hip replacement for osteoarthritis. The patient recovers from the hip pain within 3 months, but at least 1 year is required to obtain the full functional benefits of the hip replacement. Open symbols represent pain, filled symbols represent function. Circles show patients older than 72 years (*n* = 59), triangles show patients 72 years and younger (*n* = 65). Average values and 95% confidence intervals. From Nilsdotter *et al.*,[39] with permission

Currently used knee prostheses and results

Arthroplasty of the inner or outer joint compartment in the knee (most commonly medial-compartment arthroplasty) is appropriate for patients with OA in only one joint compartment, and who are over 60 years of age (Figure 7.9). This age limit, however, is only approximate, and the recommendation is based on the documented poorer results (higher frequency of revision operations) recorded for patients under 60–65 years of age who have undergone arthroplastic surgery of the knee. This higher frequency of prosthetic loosening and re-operation is probably linked to the greater demands and stresses to which younger patients expose their knees. The fraction of knee arthroplasties for OA performed with unicondylar implants varies from country to country;[41] in Sweden it is high (approximately one-fifth).[42,43]

Surgical intervention in single-compartment operations is minimal, the hospital stay short and rehabilitation less demanding for patients than for multiple-compartment surgery or osteotomy. Thus, this intervention has very few absolute contraindications from a general medical point of view. The revision rate is higher than for total knee prostheses, but a unicondylar implant can be successfully exchanged for a total knee replacement should the need arise.

Advanced or generalized OA of the knee is preferably treated with tricompartmental (total) knee prosthesis (Figure 7.10). Both smooth and porous-coated femoral implants are used. A polyethylene patellar component can be fitted, but the need for this is debated.[44] The surgery can be carried out even on very

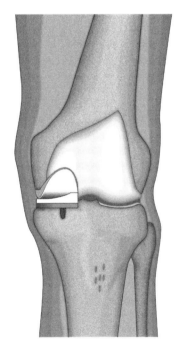

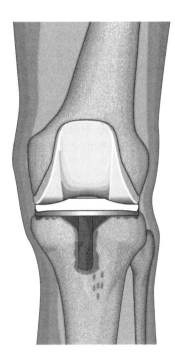

Figure 7.9 Unicompartmental (medial) knee prosthesis with a metal femoral component and a metal-backed polyethylene tibial component for use in single-compartment osteoarthritis. From *Osteoarthritis*, 2nd edn. Oxford University Press, 2003, with permission

Figure 7.10 Total (tricompartmental) knee prosthesis with a cemented metal tibial tray, which holds a modular polyethylene articulating surface. Soft-tissue tension can be adjusted by changing the thickness of the plastic component. From *Osteoarthritis*, 2nd edn. Oxford University Press, 2003, with permission

advanced OA with severe destruction of the joint. As with single-compartment arthroplasty, the prosthesis is more likely to come loose in younger patients, so the benefits of joint-replacement surgery in those younger than about 60 years will need to be balanced against this risk.[42,43,45] The surgical intervention and rehabilitation may be more demanding for the patient than single-compartment arthroplasty. For seriously overweight patients, the surgery may be more difficult, but even in these patients, the results have proven to be good. There is no need for an upper age limit; results are good even among the eldest patients. The results of knee arthroplasty have been followed-up continuously for more than 20 years and reported to the national Swedish knee register. During this time period, the results have gradually improved and are now at least as good as those of hip arthroplasty. Loosening of the prosthesis and wear of the prosthetic components remains a problem, as is the case for the replaced hip, but even 10 years after the operation more than 90% of patients have a knee that works well.[46]

The surgical treatment of isolated patellofemoral OA remains a problem; a review of the literature provides conflicting evidence of the benefits of surgery, including endoprosthetic replacement of the patella.

Patients who undergo joint-replacement surgery should be aware that they will get a new knee, but not a normal knee. The joint becomes stable and pain-free with good mobility, which allows ordinary daily activities such as walking, cycling, swimming and other light exercise or work. Strong physical exertion is not recommended, and the patient should be advised against heavy work with strain on the knee, owing to the risk of the prosthesis working loose.

Sales statistics in Europe show that three-quarters of tibial components are cemented, while cementless femoral fixation is slightly more common than cemented.

Arthroplasties of the ankle, shoulder, elbow and hand

Symptomatic OA of the ankle is uncommon and often secondary to deformity, joint instability, ankle fracture or vascular necrosis of the talus. A common surgical treatment is ankle fusion (arthrodesis). In patients aged over 60 years with limited expectations on physical activity, and without instability, deformity or neuropathic disorders, an ankle arthroplasty may be considered. A variety of implants have been designed, but reports on outcome are few and short term.

OA of the shoulder is not the most common indication for shoulder arthroplasty, a procedure constituting 1% of all large-joint arthroplasties. As with the ankle, reports on outcome are few and short term.

Symptomatic OA of the elbow is a rare condition, and more than 95% of all elbow arthroplasties are performed for other indications.

OA of the fingers affects both the proximal and distal joints. The initially painful arthritis and joint degeneration eventually cause stiff, slightly deformed but stable joints that need not be treated with implants, although they are available for rheumatoid arthritis. The saddle-shaped trapeziometacarpal joint of the thumb is a common location for OA of the hand. Every fourth woman will develop some joint degeneration, with 1 in 20 being a candidate for surgery.[13] Surgical treatment includes partial or total excision of the trapezium with ligament reconstruction and interposition of tendinous structures or a silicone implant.

Arthroplasty complications

The prevalence of symptomatic OA increases with age, as do the risks of general complications due to major surgery. Improvements in risk assessment and anaesthesiological technique have made it possible to offer arthroplasty even to the very old. With modern hip arthroplasty technique and hypotensive epidural anaesthesia, the mortality rate is in the order of 0.1%.[47,48] The risk of deep-vein thrombosis and pulmonary embolism is significantly reduced by the use of epidural, rather than general, anaesthesia, compression stockings, foot compression pumps and early ambulation, as well as pharmacological prophylaxis with low molecular-weight heparin or other antithrombotic agents. The best prevention against complications is a properly selected, well-informed, well-nourished, well-monitored patient, who has replacement of blood loss and who is pain-free. Recognition of the importance of being pain-free has led to changes in post-operative routines, including continued epidural analgesia, personally adjusted doses and post-operative self-administration of morphine.

Hip arthroplasty

Early, local post-operative complications include delayed wound healing, deep infection, dislocation, avulsion of the greater trochanter and pseudarthrosis of a trochanteric osteotomy. Dislocation has been reported in 0.5–5% of patients. The joint can usually be reduced, and the problem may resolve as a pseudocapsule develops around it. Dislocation is associated with prior surgery of the hip, use of a posterior approach and malaligned components.[49] Trochanteric problems are reported with the same frequency and to these should be added the formation of heterotopic bone; when pronounced, it may reduce mobility.

Loosening of implant components is the indication for 80% of hip revisions. Deep infection is a serious complication. Three types are encountered: early and delayed post-operative, and late haematogenous, i.e. bacterial seeding from some other focus, such as the urinary tract, gall bladder, lungs or a dental abscess. Typically, the patient is not pain-free, the erythrocyte sedimentation rate remains elevated and, sometimes, low-grade fever is noted. Wound healing may be disturbed or a fistula may develop. Radiographic examination may show rapid loosening of the components. For the majority of deep infections, the only safe method is removal of the implant. Modern two-stage revision techniques include extraction of the prosthesis, a 6-week period with gentamicin-containing cement beads or a gentamicin-containing bone cement 'spacer' inserted in the bone defect, antibiotic treatment, and re-implantation of a new prosthesis. The overall success rate is in the range of 75–95%.

The risk of a late, deep implant infection is increased in connection with e.g. urosepsis, 'dirty' surgery or dental root canal procedures. Antibiotic prophylaxis is recommended in connection with such procedures, but not with routine dental work, such as fillings.

Knee arthroplasty

The knee may have undergone surgery before arthroplasty, which may increase the risk of conflicting skin incisions, with healing disturbances and a high risk of deep infection.

Loosening of components, mainly the tibial, is the indication in half of all knee arthroplasty revisions. In total knee arthroplasty for OA, the cumulative risk of revision for loosening is 3% at 10 years. This low level has been reached by improvements in instrumentation, prosthetic design and cementation technique. For unicompartmental implants, the risk of loosening is twice as high. The best revision results are achieved if a new total knee implant is used with exchange of all components.

Delayed or late infection may present as chronic arthritis, with fibrosis and joint contracture. Eventually the implants become loose. Late infection can also occur as an abscess or a fistula. Usually, the bone–cement interface is also infected, and revision is needed. The cumulative risk of revision for deep infection is less than 1% at 10 years. Half of the revisions are performed as one- or two-stage exchange arthroplasties, and the remainder as knee fusions.

The Scandinavian national arthroplasty registers

In 1975, the Swedish Orthopaedic Society initiated a prospective nationwide register of knee arthroplasty.[50–52] It was followed by a national hip arthroplasty register in 1979.[53,54] Other Scandinavian countries subsequently started similar registers.[55–57] These registers use social-security numbers to keep track of all patients. Individual patient mortality can be checked against national census registers, and arthroplasty registers can be linked to many other population-based registers. Data are regularly analysed by actuarial methods, to calculate the cumulated risk of revision for various groups of patients, implants and surgical techniques, and results are posted on the Internet.[37,58]

The results from these nationwide registers cover more than 90% of all primary arthroplasties and revisions, and provide population-based and more realistic assessments of results and risks than reports from highly specialized units. The registers have identified inferior arthroplasty designs, prompting their removal from the market. They have also shown that the modern, conventional, cemented implants have been and remain a safe choice.

The original arthroplasty registers, by design, focused on revision, but not all revisions are equal, and clinical, patient-relevant performance was not taken into account.[59] More recently, aspects of outcome other than re-operation have been introduced in the registries.[37,46] Joint-replacement registries are now being established in an increasing number of countries, facilitating international comparisons of usage and outcome.[60–64]

References

1. Buckwalter JA, Lohmander S. Operative treatment of osteoarthrosis: current practice and future development. J Bone Joint Surg 1994; 76A: 1405–18

2. Buckwalter JA, Lohmander LS. Surgical approaches to preserving and restoring articular cartilage. In Brandt KD, Doherty M, Lohmander LS, eds. Osteoarthritis, 2nd edn. Oxford: Oxford University Press, 2003: 353–60

3. Bert JM. Role of abrasion arthroplasty and debridement in the management of osteoarthritis of the knee. Rheum Dis Clin North Am 1993; 19: 725–39

4.   Bert JM, Maschka K. The arthroscopic treatment of unicompartmental gonarthrosis. Arthroscopy 1989; 5: 25–32

5.   Dandy DJ. Arthroscopic debridement of the knee for osteoarthritis. J Bone Joint Surg 1991; 73B: 877–8

6.   Johnson LL. Diagnostic and surgical arthroscopy. St Louis: CV Mosby, 1980

7.   Hubbard MJS. Arthroscopic surgery for chondral flaps in the knee. J Bone Joint Surg 1987; 69B: 794–6

8.   Gibson JNA, Whit MD, Chapman VM, Strachan RK. Arthroscopic lavage and debridement for osteoarthritis of the knee. J Bone Joint Surg 1992; 74B: 534–7

9.   Livesley PJ, Doherty M, Needoff M, Moulton A. Arthroscopic lavage of osteoarthritic knees. J Bone Joint Surg 1991; 73B: 922–6

10. Moseley JB, O'Malley K, Petersen NJ, et al. A controlled trial of arthroscopic surgery for osteoarthritis of the knee. N Engl J Med 2002; 347: 81–8

11. Shapiro F, Koide S, Glimcher MJ. Cell origin and differentiation in the repair of full-thickness defects of articular cartilage. J Bone Joint Surg 1993; 75A: 532–53

12. Campbell II DC. Arthroplasty of the metatarsophalangeal joint. In Morrey BM, ed. Joint replacement arthroplasty. Rochester: Churchill Livingstone, 1991: 1183–92

13. Cooney WP. Arthroplasty of the thumb axis. In Morrey BM, ed. Joint replacement arthroplasty. Rochester: Churchill Livingstone, 1991: 173–94

14. Hangody L, Feczko P, Bartha L, et al. Mosaicplasty for the treatment of articular defects of the knee and ankle. Clin Orthop 2001; 391 (Suppl): S328–36

15. Brittberg M, Lindahl A, Nilsson A, et al. Treatment of deep cartilage defects in the knee with autologous chondrocyte transplantation. N Engl J Med 1994; 331: 889–95

16. Peterson L, Brittberg M, Kiviranta I, et al. Autologous chondrocyte transplantation. Biomechanics and long-term durability. Am J Sports Med 2002; 30: 2–12

17. Lohmander LS. Cell-based cartilage repair – do we need it, can we do it, is it good, can we prove it? Curr Opin Orthop 1998; 9: 38–42

18. Bergenudd H, Johnell O, Redlund-Johnell I, Lohmander LS. The articular cartilage after osteotomy for medial gonarthrosis: biopsies after 2 years in 19 cases. Acta Orthop Scand 1992; 63: 413–16

19. Odenbring S, Egund N, Lindstrand A, et al. Cartilage regeneration after proximal tibial osteotomy for medial gonarthrosis. Clin Orthop 1992; 277: 210–16

20. Itoman M, Yamamoto M, Yonemoto K, et al. Histological examination of surface repair tissue after successful osteotomy for osteoarthritis of the hip. Int Orthop (Germany) 1992; 16: 118–21

21. Insall JN, Joseph DM, Msika C. High tibial osteotomy for varus gonarthrosis. A long-term follow-up study. J Bone Joint Surg 1984; 66A: 1040–8

22. Reigstad A, Gronmark T. Osteoarthritis of the hip treated by intertrochanteric osteotomy. A long-term follow up. J Bone Joint Surg 1984; 66A: 1–6

23. Berman AT, Bosco SJ, Kirshner S, Avolio A. Factors influencing long-term results in high tibial osteotomy. Clin Orthop 1991; 272: 192–8

24. Coventry MB, Ilstrup DM, Wallrichs SL. Proximal tibial osteotomy. A critical long-term study of eighty-seven cases. J Bone Joint Surg 1993; 75A: 196–201

25. Odenbring S, Tjornstrand B, Egund N, et al. Function after tibial osteotomy for medial gonarthrosis below aged 50 years. Acta Ortho Scand 1989; 60: 527–31

26. Odenbring S, Egund N, Knutson K, et al. Revision after osteotomy for gonarthrosis. A 10–19 year follow-up of 314 cases. Acta Orthop Scand 1990; 61: 128–30

27. Weidenhielm L, Olsson E, Brostrom LA, et al. Improvement in gait one year after surgery for knee osteoarthrosis: a comparison between high tibial osteotomy and prosthetic replacement in a prospective randomized study. Scand J Rehabil Med 1993; 25: 25–31

28. Magyar G, Ahl TL, Vibe P, et al. Open-wedge osteotomy by hemicallotasis or the closed-wedge technique for osteoarthritis of the knee. A randomised study of 50 operations. J Bone Joint Surg 1999; 81: 444–8

29. Hadorn DC, Holmes AC. The New Zealand priority criteria project. Part 1: Overview. Br Med J 1997; 314: 131–4

30. Hadorn D. Steering Committee of the Western Canada Waiting List Project. Setting priorities on waiting lists: point-count systems as linear models. J Health Serv Res Policy 2003; 8: 48–54

31. Hawker GA, Wright JG, Glazier RH, et al. The effect of education and income on need and willingness to undergo total joint arthroplasty. Arthritis Rheum 2002; 46: 3331–9

32. Juni P, Dieppe P, Donovan J, et al. Population requirement for primary knee replacement surgery: a cross-sectional study. Rheumatology (Oxford) 2003; 42: 516–21

33. Waugh W. John Charnley. The man and the hip. London: Springer-Verlag, 1990

34. Rothman RC, Cohn JC. Cemented versus cementless total hip arthroplasty: a critical review. Clin Orthop 1990; 254: 153–69

35. Huiskes R. Failed innovation in total hip replacement. Diagnosis and proposals for a cure. Acta Orthop Scand 1993; 64: 699–716

36. Malchau H, Herberts P, Ahnfelt L. Prognosis of total hip replacement in Sweden: follow-up of 92,675 operations performed 1978–1990. Acta Orthop Scand 1993; 64: 497–506

37. http://www.jru.orthop.gu.se/ (Accessed June 2004)

38. Havelin LI, Espehaug B, Vollset SE, Engesæter LB. Early failures among 14,009 cemented and 1,326 uncemented prostheses for primary coxarthrosis: the Norwegian Arthroplasty Register 1987–1992. Acta Orthop Scand 1994; 65: 1–6

39. Nilsdotter A-K, Lohmander LS. Age and waiting time as predictors for outcome after total hip replacement for osteoarthritis. Rheumatology 2002; 41: 1261–7

40. Nilsdotter A-K, Petersson IF, Roos EM, Lohmander LS. Predictors of patient-relevant outcome after total hip replacement for osteoarthritis – a prospective study. Ann Rheum Dis 2003; 62: 923–30

41. Grelsamer RP. Current concepts review. Unicompartmental osteoarthrosis of the knee. J Bone Joint Surg 1995; 77A: 278–92

42. Knutson K, Lindstrand L, Lidgren L. Survival of knee arthroplasties. A nation-wide multicentre investigation of 8000 cases. J Bone Joint Surg 1986; 68B: 795–803

43. Robertsson O, Knutson K, Lewold S, Lidgren L. The Swedish Knee Arthroplasty Register 1975–1997. An update with special emphasis on 41,223 knees operated on in 1988–1997. Acta Orthop Scand 2001; 72: 503–13

44. Rand JA. Current concepts review. The patellofemoral joint in total knee arthroplasty. J Bone Joint Surg 1994; 76A: 612–20

45. Harrysson OL, Robertsson O, Nayfeh JF. Higher cumulative revision rate of knee arthroplasties in younger patients with osteoarthritis. Clin Orthop 2004; 421: 162–8

46. Robertsson O, Dunbar MJ. Patient satisfaction compared with general health and disease-specific questionnaires in knee arthroplasty patients. J Arthroplasty 2001; 16: 476–82

47. Sharrock NE, Cazan MG, Hargett MJL, et al. Changes in mortality after hip and knee arthroplasty over a ten-year period. Anesthesia Analgesia 1995; 80: 242–8

48. Lie SA, Engesaeter LB, Havelin LI, et al. Early postoperative mortality after 67,548 total hip replacements: causes of death and thromboprophylaxis in 68 hospitals in Norway from 1987 to 1999. Acta Orthop Scand 2002; 73: 392–9

49. Morrey BF. Instability after total hip arthroplasty. Orthop Clinics North Am 1992; 23: 237–48

50. Knutson K, Lindstrand L, Lidgren L. Survival of knee arthroplasties. A nation-wide multicentre investigation of 8000 cases. J Bone Joint Surg 1986; 68-B: 795–803

51. Knutson K, Lewold S, Robertsson O, Lidgren L. The Swedish Knee Arthroplasty Register. A nation-wide study of 30,003 knees 1976–1992. Acta Orthop Scand 1994; 65: 375–86

52. Robertsson O, Knutson K, Lewold S, Lidgren L. The Swedish Knee Arthroplasty Register 1975–1997. An update with special emphasis on 41,223 knees operated on in 1988–1997. Acta Orthop Scand 2001; 72: 503–13

53. Malchau H, Herberts P, Ahnfelt L. Prognosis of total hip replacement in Sweden: follow-up of 92,675 operations performed 1978–1990. Acta Orthop Scand 1993; 64: 497–506

54. Malchau H, Herberts P, Eisler T, et al. The Swedish Total Hip Replacement Register. J Bone Joint Surg 2002; 84-A (Suppl 2): 2–20

55. Espehaug B, Havelin LI, Engesæter LB, et al. Early revision among 12,179 hip prostheses. A comparison of 10 different brands reported to the Norwegian Arthroplasty Register, 1987–1993. Acta Orthop Scand 1995; 66: 487–93

56. Havelin LI, Espehaug B, Vollset SE, et al. The Norwegian arthroplasty register: a survey of 17,444 hip replacements 1987–1990. Acta Orthop Scand 1993; 64: 245–51

57. Havelin LI, Vollset SE, Engesæter LB. Revision for aseptic loosening of uncemented cups in 4352 primary total hip prostheses: a report from the Arthroplasty Register. Acta Orthop Scand 1995; 66: 494–500

58. http://www.ort.lu.se/knee/indexeng.html (Accessed June 2004)

59. Britton AR, Murray DW, Bulstrode CJ, et al. Pain levels after total hip replacement: their use as endpoints for survival analysis. J Bone Joint Surg 1997; 79B: 93–8

60. http://info.haukeland.no/nrl/ (Accessed June 2004)

61. http://www.dmac.adelaide.edu.au/aoanjrr/index.jsp (Accessed June 2004)

62. http://www.cdhb.govt.nz/NJR/ (Accessed June 2004)

63. http://secure.cihi.ca/cihiweb/dispPage.jsp?cw_page=services_cjrr_e (Accessed June 2004)

64. http://www.njrcentre.org.uk/ (Accessed June 2004)

8

Management of osteoarthritis

Paul Creamer

INTRODUCTION

Previous chapters have considered in detail the surgical and non-surgical treatment of osteoarthritis (OA). This chapter will discuss how such treatments can be unified into a general management approach, with particular emphasis on the patient's perspective.

OA is the most common disease to affect synovial joints, and the single most important cause of disability and handicap from arthritis. Knee OA is strongly associated with ageing and obesity, and therefore represents an increasing burden on Western health-care systems. Pathologically, OA is associated with loss of articular cartilage, osteophyte formation, changes in subchondral bone, thickening of joint capsule, muscle changes and variable degrees of synovitis. Some of these changes result in typical radiographic features of joint-space narrowing, osteophyte formation and subchondral sclerosis.

Most data on the management of peripheral joint OA focus on the knee, though it seems likely that the general management principles will hold for the other common joint sites (hip, hand). There are good reasons for the knee to assume predominance: 5–15% of people aged 35–74 years have radiographic evidence[1] of knee OA; of these, perhaps 50% will be symptomatic. About 25% of subjects aged 60 years or above complain of knee pain, of whom half have associated disability. In a typical UK or USA population, for every 100 000 individuals, 7500 will have knee pain and disability due to OA, 2000 of whom have severe disability[2]. Clearly, the burden of such a prevalent condition falls mainly on primary care, and management should be focused on the community rather than the hospital.

Not all individuals with knee pain seek medical attention, even those with severely painful and disabling symptoms. The reasons why some individuals elect to seek care are unclear, but probably do not simply reflect disease severity. Other reasons may include any of the following:

(1)   Sudden worsening of symptoms;

(2)   Socio-economic or work factors;

(3)   Co-morbidity;

(4)   Cultural expectations;

(5)   Coping strategies;

(6)   Availability of services.

When considering the management of OA, it is helpful to use the International Classification of Function (ICF) model. Thus, OA may result in 'Impairment' (for example, the inability to bend the knee fully), which may in turn cause 'Activity Limitation' (unable to get into and out of a car), which in turn results in 'Participation Restriction' (unable to drive to shops). To these three categories may be added 'Mood' (anxiety, depression, helplessness). Implicit in this model is the concept of 'Individualization'; the development of a treatment strategy for each patient should be based on their particular needs and expectations as well as the evidence base. The aims of managing OA may be summarized as:

(1)   Educating patients and carers;

(2)   Alleviating pain;

(3)   Improving disability, activity restriction and non-participation;

(4)   Reducing progression.

Central to provision of this care is a 'team' approach involving health-care professionals and the patient, to develop a package of care tailored to the individual.

DIAGNOSIS AND DEFINITION

OA may be viewed as having three components, each with separate risk factors: pain, disability and structural change. Management of one may have no effect on the others. OA may be defined in terms of symptoms, radiographic change or pathology; these may overlap but frequently do not.

Pathological data are, in general, unavailable. Unfortunately, X-rays are a poor surrogate for pathological change as early changes (which may be confirmed by arthroscopy or magnetic resonance imaging) are not observed on X-ray. A normal X-ray, therefore, does not exclude OA. Although for epidemiological studies it has been suggested that OA should be defined by symptoms (usually pain) plus evidence of structural change (usually X-ray change), this would exclude individuals with early OA and normal X-rays.

The American College of Rheumatology Classification Criteria for knee OA include knee pain and age over 40 years, with morning stiffness persisting less than 30 minutes and crepitus on motion.[3] A reasonable working diagnostic approach to OA is to assume that knee pain over the age of 50 years is due to OA, unless another cause can be found, especially if pain is worse on use, and associated with stiffness after inactivity and restricted movement. In practice, it may be more helpful, therefore, to consider management of 'knee pain' or 'hip pain', rather than OA. Table 8.1 indicates the typical features of OA and some of the alternative diagnoses that should be excluded at the hip and knee.

Radiographs are frequently requested, and are useful in confirming that established OA is present and in defining which joints (or parts of joints) are affected. Taken serially, they also allow assessment of progression. They are also of value in excluding other causes of joint pain, for example fracture, avascular necrosis and Paget's disease. Radiographs are not useful in diagnosing early

Table 8.1 Clinical and differential diagnosis of knee and hip osteoarthritis (OA)

Typical features suggesting OA	Pain – deep, poorly localized, worse on use	
	Stiffness – localized to involved joints, rarely exceeds 30 minutes	
	Crepitus on active motion	
	Limited range of movement	
	No systemic features	
Differential diagnoses to consider	*Knee*	*Hip*
Other arthritis	RA, gout, CPPD	RA, seronegative spondarthropathy
Bone disease	Avascular necrosis Paget's disease	Avascular necrosis Paget's disease
Soft tissue	Meniscal or ligament injuries	Bursitis, tendinopathy
Referred pain	From hip	From spine, SIJ

RA, rheumatoid arthritis; CPPD, calcium pyrophosphate deposition; SIJ, sacroiliac joint

disease (often normal even when pathology is present), nor can they indicate the impact of disease on the individual or allow a prognosis to be made. Possible indications for obtaining an X-ray in a patient with knee pain might be:

(1)   Knee pain that suddenly gets worse;

(2)   Acute inflammation or other signs that suggest a diagnosis other than OA (Table 8.1);

(3)   Possible referral from hip;

(4)   Investigation prior to surgery.

HOW DOES OSTEOARTHRITIS AFFECT THE PATIENT?

For a logical approach to management to be established, it is necessary to understand the impact of OA on affected individuals.

Pain and stiffness

In many cases, OA is asymptomatic; up to 40% of individuals with severe radiographic knee OA do not report pain. Pain-free individuals are unlikely to ever present to medical care, and management of OA is therefore based on symptomatic individuals (probably representing a minority of the total 'disease'). When OA does cause symptoms, pain is most frequently reported and is the principal reason why individuals elect to seek medical care. Pain is also one of the major determinants of functional loss. Pain in OA may be as severe as that of rheumatoid arthritis, though there is large variability ('good days and bad days') influenced by activity, climatic conditions, season and co-morbidity. A diurnal variation exists in most patients, with pain being better in the morning and worse in the evening. When considering the management of pain it is helpful to remember the biopsychosocial model (Figure 8.1), emphasizing that the subjective experience of pain is modulated by many factors other than current structural disease.[4]

Disability

Symptomatic knee OA is associated with self-reported disability, particularly for activities involving mobility and transfer, and instrumental activities of daily living.[5] Risk factors include pain, low educational status, obesity, female gender,

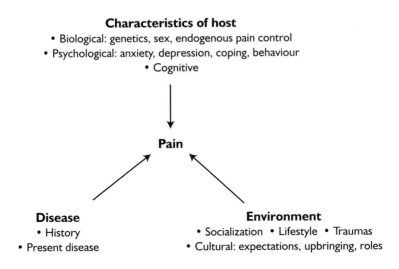

Figure 8.1 Biopsychosocial factors that interact and modulate the experience of pain (reproduced with permission from Holdcroft 2003[4])

age and quadriceps weakness. Structural change by X-ray is only weakly related to disability, though the relationship may vary with disease duration. van Baar *et al.*, studying community dwellers with a shorter (median 65 weeks) duration of OA, reported significant correlation between structural change and disability.[2] It may be that with chronicity other factors such as coping skills and social support are more important than structural change in determining the level of disability.

Psychological impact

OA may be associated with less depression than other musculoskeletal disorders such as rheumatoid arthritis but, as with most chronic diseases, patients with OA have higher depression rates than the general population. A study of 463 outpatients with hip or knee OA[6] found 'possible depression' in 33%, compared with a population prevalence of 19%. Depression may have a role in promoting health-care-seeking behaviour by patients; a community study of individuals with symptomatic hip or knee OA found depression scores to be significantly higher in those subjects who had elected to seek medical care.[7] OA may result in other psychological changes, such as anxiety and 'loss of control', a result of pain and activity restriction.

General health status, participation and quality of life

Compared with controls matched for age, gender and residential community, subjects with symptomatic OA experience losses in the performance of house-hold chores, shopping, errands and leisure activities, and spend more time sleeping and engaged in personal hygiene.[8] The impact of OA may be greater in younger patients than old. De Bock *et al.*[9] used the Sickness Impact Profile to assess the impact of OA on a community group, compared with matched controls. Impairment of ambulation, body care and movement, emotional behaviour, sleep and rest, home management and work was seen in subjects aged 41–60 years. In subjects aged 61–75 years, differences were only seen in emotional, sleep and work domains. Clearly, knee OA in a 75-year-old woman has a different meaning than the same disease in a 50-year-old with a job and lifestyle contingent on physical mobility. An elderly person may view chronic disease such as OA as an expected consequence of the ageing process.[10,11]

Patients awaiting hip replacement for OA are more likely to be restricted in their physical and social life than matched controls, but mental state and vitality remain unimpaired. Lower social class adds to the burden on health status, particularly social functioning.[12]

GUIDELINES FOR MANAGING OSTEOARTHRITIS

Several guidelines for the management of lower-limb OA have been produced, usually as consensus statements from expert panels.[13–16] The European League against Rheumatism (EULAR) 2000 recommendations are unusual in that they include indications of the level of evidence to support individual statements.[15] These guidelines provide a good summary of the evidence base underlying non-surgical interventions, but their use in daily practice is limited by several factors:

(1) By definition they can only evaluate available data, which for some interventions (especially physical), are sparse. Most published research has examined drugs (59%) or surgery (27%).[17] Moreover, most (94%) report positive results, suggesting a bias against publishing negative findings. The EULAR guidelines[15] reviewed 674 papers, of which 564 concerned drug or

surgical therapy (of which 365 involved non-steroidal anti-inflammatory drugs (NSAIDs)).

(2)   Recommendations made in guidelines may not be practical, due to local constraints or lack of resources.

(3)   Guidelines do not distinguish between the provision of primary and secondary care.

(4)   The guidelines are designed to be applied to groups of patients, whereas an individualized approach to management is likely to be more effective. Clearly, the need for weight reduction, for example, is greater in some patients than others.

(5)   In practice, treatments are rarely applied sequentially; rather, combinations of interventions are applied simultaneously. The effect of such 'packages' of care is unknown.

It is also true that, despite good evidence for many non-surgical treatments in OA, most patients remain under-managed, and significant improvement could be made simply by making better use of the therapies currently available.

Table 8.2 indicates the issues that should be considered when planning treatment. The age of the patient is probably the least important, but may affect the decision to consider surgery (though how age affects this decision is unclear). Surgeons may prefer to operate on older people, reducing the chances of having to perform difficult revision surgery in the future; patients themselves may feel that younger, more active individuals should have the chance of total joint replacement (TJR). Co-morbidity should be considered. Does the patient have contraindications to the use of NSAIDs? Does the patient have cardiovascular disease limiting mobility more than the OA? Would the patient have a high operative risk if TJR were to be considered? Risk factors for OA should be assessed: Is the patient obese? Are they at risk of occupational overuse?

Table 8.2 Considerations when planning the management of patients with osteoarthritis (OA)

Age
Co-morbidities
Risk factors
Impact of OA
Individual preference
Availability of services

Are there psychosocial factors that may confer a worse prognosis? The impact of OA should be assessed using the ICF model, including pain severity, impairment of function and the effect of this on the individual.

The patient's preference for treatment should be explored and attempts should be made to identify the issues that are of importance to that individual. The treatment plan should be developed through a dynamic partnership between patient and doctor. Finally, management is necessarily affected by local service provision, such as length of waiting list, access to physiotherapy, etc.

MINIMUM CARE PACKAGE

Given the variability introduced by the factors described above, it is rarely practical to follow the standard sequential approach to managing patients advocated by guidelines. For all individuals with OA electing to seek medical care, a minimum care package should be offered, including education, exercise, advice on weight reduction, correction of adverse mechanics and advice on the use of simple analgesics.

Education

Education is particularly important in OA, where much depends on the patient assuming control for their own care. It should aim to dispel myths such as the inevitability of OA or that 'nothing will help', and provide information on disease process, likely outcome, available treatments (and how to use them) and lifestyle adaptations to the disease. The effect of education by itself on important outcomes such as pain appears to be relatively weak; one study showed that only 38% of patients found education moderately or very helpful.[18] More remains to be learnt about how and when to deliver education packages, but it may be that education allows a reduction in perceived helplessness, disability and impact, rather than pain.

Exercise

Exercise may be divided into specific muscle strengthening exercises (e.g. quadriceps for knee) and graded aerobic exercise programmes. Advice on simple walking programmes and basic quadriceps exercises can be delivered at home and should form part of the 'basic package'.

Weight reduction

Obesity is an important risk factor for OA; subjects who lose weight are less likely to progress radiographically or develop symptoms.[19] Proving that weight loss reduces pain levels is difficult, largely because of the problems in achieving significant weight reduction. Moreover, weight reduction is often combined with exercise, which itself has an effect on the symptoms of OA. More remains to be learnt about the best ways of encouraging weight loss; different approaches may be effective in different individuals. Nevertheless, weight reduction is a powerful disease-modifying intervention that deserves intensive effort in all obese patients with lower-limb OA.

Biomechanical approaches

Comfortable shoes with shock-absorbing insoles can reduce knee pain in OA. Heel wedges are a method of correcting the abnormal biomechanics seen in knee OA. A laterally elevated (valgus) insole may decrease lateral thrust and reduce pain in subjects with medial-compartment OA. Knee braces are sometimes used to correct deformity and reduce pain. Provision of a cane or walking stick may reduce pain and improve function by 'unloading' the joint.

Medication

Patients should be informed about drug options, but many may choose not to use drugs. It should be made clear to patients that drugs are purely for symptom relief and that it is entirely reasonable, if patients prefer, to put up with the pain rather than take medication. If medication is required, paracetamol (acetaminophen) remains the drug of choice. Topical anti-inflammatory creams and gels are useful for small-joint OA, and have the advantage of safety and giving the patient some control over how and when they treat themselves. Many patients will seek alternative or complementary medications; this popular approach should be discussed and patients directed to those supplements for which some evidence exists (e.g. chondroitin, unsaturated oils).

Treatment beyond this basic package depends on the many variables mentioned above, but any of the options in Table 8.3 can be considered. A number of scenarios may be envisaged – representative case studies are presented in Table 8.4, in approximately ascending order of severity.

Table 8.3 Therapeutic options in osteoarthritis

Education	Patient and spouse or family
Weight loss	
Social support	Telephone contact, helplines, support groups, formal cognitive interventions
Exercise	Muscle strengthening, patellar strapping, aerobic exercise (walking, swimming, cycling)
Orthotics and footwear	Aids and appliances, joint protection, insoles
Dietary supplements	Glucosamine, vitamins C and D, ginger, avocado and soybean extracts, fish oils
Topical drugs	Topical NSAIDs, rubifacients, capsaicin
Oral drugs	Analgesics (paracetamol, codydramol, opiates), NSAIDs, cyclo-oxygenase-2 selective NSAIDs
Intra-articular treatment	Corticosteroids, hyaluronans
Surgical interventions	Tidal lavage and debridement, osteotomy, total joint arthroplasty
Other	Acupuncture, TENS

NSAIDs, non-steroidal anti-inflammatory drugs; TENS, transcutaneous electrical nerve stimulation

Case 1: Mild osteoarthritis

Basic package as outlined above. X-rays are not indicated. 'Medicalization' should be avoided if possible. The concept of gradual joint failure with a variety of outcomes is preferable to a 'disease' label.

Case 2: Moderate OA, no other problems

Basic package as outlined above. This patient will probably need analgesia. If paracetamol is inadequate, a stronger analgesia (codydramol, coproxamol, tramadol) should be tried. If these fail, a trial of an NSAID should be performed. The patient should be reassessed at 1 month and the additional benefit of the NSAID over and above that of analgesia should be evaluated. The minimum effective dose should be used and, wherever possible, the patient should be instructed to take the NSAID in short courses (for 'flare-ups') rather than continuously. Traditional NSAIDs have a high risk of side-effects. The introduction of COX2 inhibitors with a better theoretical safety profile has led to suggestions that these drugs be used as first-line therapy, before analgesics and

Table 8.4 Representative osteoarthritis (OA) case studies

Case 1: Mild OA

Mrs Smith is a 68-year-old woman with a 2-year history of bilateral knee pain. She is otherwise fit and well. The knee pain does not concern her greatly; indeed, she describes it as an 'ache' rather than pain. She lives independently and enjoys gardening. She is slightly overweight. Her main concern is that she wants to ensure things do not get worse.

Case 2: Moderate OA, no other problems

Mr Brown is a 50-year-old accountant with a 12-month history of left hip pain. The pain is centred on the groin. It interferes with his ability to cycle to work but does not keep him awake at night. Examination shows reduced internal rotation by about 40%. He is worried because his father had a hip replacement aged 70 years.

Case 3: Moderate OA with co-morbidity

Mrs Jones is an 80-year-old woman with a 5-year history of painful interphalangeal joints. Joints seem to go through phases of pain, swelling and inflammation, eventually settling after about 6 months. She finds it hard to perform fine tasks such as doing up buttons, which is troublesome as she is a widow and lives alone. 2 years ago she was investigated for anaemia and was found to have a small gastric ulcer.

Case 4: Severe OA

Mrs Green is a 70-year-old woman with bilateral knee pain. She has pain every day and finds it difficult getting up and down stairs, in and out of cars and coping with activities of daily living. She relies on her daughter for help with cleaning and shopping. She has tried three different NSAIDs but all upset her stomach. Paracetamol is ineffective and codeine preparations make her constipated; in addition, she does not like tablets. She is overweight at 85 kg.

NSAIDs, non-steroidal anti-inflammatory drugs

traditional NSAIDs. However, the reduction in toxicity with these drugs may have been overstated, notably in elderly populations (which include most patients with OA), and concerns remain about side-effects, including cardiovascular events. Until more robust data to the contrary are available, clinical evidence continues to support the safety of paracetamol over NSAIDs.

Advice on footwear should be given. Patients with this level of symptoms may benefit from formal physiotherapy review and hydrotherapy. Local steroid injections would be very appropriate if the patient had knee or thumb base pain, but can still be undertaken at the hip under X-ray or ultrasound control.

Case 3: Moderate osteoarthritis with co-morbidity

Basic package as outlined above. In some patients, treatment of co-morbidities may result in better outcomes for the patient than treatment of the OA itself. Depression and anxiety should not be forgotten, particularly in the isolated elderly. In these cases, non-drug therapy, such as occupational therapy, specific hand therapy and advice on hot and cold relief, is as important as drugs. Systemic NSAIDs should be avoided, but topical NSAIDs and topical capsaicin would be appropriate. Local steroid injections to the thumb base are often helpful (less so to interphalangeal joints).

Case 4: Severe osteoarthritis

Basic package as above. An aggressive approach to management is indicated, with prompt referral to physiotherapy, trial of local steroid injections (at least twice) and support for weight reduction. Opiates are probably underused in OA, though they are effective. Concerns about patient addiction and vulnerability to legal action has led physicians to be reluctant to prescribe these drugs. In fact, addiction rates in otherwise psychologically stable individuals are very low. Reluctance to use powerful opiates is one example of the discrepancy that may exist between patients and doctors in analysing the risk–benefit trade-off of interventions – doctors perceive their patients to be less badly off than patients perceive themselves; as a result, patients are willing to accept greater risks to achieve pain reduction. If these measures fail, then total knee replacement (TKR) should be considered.

WHO CURRENTLY GETS TOTAL JOINT REPLACEMENT?

OA is the main disease leading to total hip replacement (THR) or TKR, accounting for about 80% of such operations.[20,21] Current rates of joint replacement vary greatly between different countries. Rates for THR in Organisation for Economic Co-operation and Development (OECD) countries range from 50 to 130/100 000 population.[22] Sweden has the highest rate of THR and the US the highest rate of TKR. To some extent, this may reflect different coding systems and prevalence rates of OA, but it may also be due to different socio-economic factors, population age structures, health-care systems and indications for TJR. Even within the UK there are large (threefold) variations in the rates of THR between different regions.

Hospital episode statistics[23] indicate that between 1991 and 2000 the rate of primary THR in the UK increased from 65.5 to 77.6/100 000. Increases were especially seen in older people, but there was a doubling in the rate of revision surgery – more expensive and technically more difficult – to 19.2/100 000. The rate of TKR in the UK is lower but increasing rapidly, doubling from 32.8 to 66.8/100 000 in the last 10 years; thus, TKR is set to become more common than THR (already the case in the US). These figures are derived from the National Health Service (NHS); the figure including operations performed in the private sector is probably about 20% higher. The need for TJR is likely to increase by about 30% in the next 30 years, largely due to an ageing population.

Women tend to have worse function at the time of surgery than men. American data suggest that elderly, obese and black populations are less likely to obtain a TJR than middle-aged, middle-class whites, despite the fact that there is no evidence that older obese patients have worse outcomes. UK studies confirm that social deprivation reduces the chance of having a TJR.[21]

A recent study from France[24] of 772 patients with knee OA found a 2-year TKR rate of 9.5%. Risk factors for TKR included pain (area under curve (AUC) highest tertile vs. lowest odds ratio (OR) 3.5; $p = 0.0002$) and X-ray severity (Kellgren and Lawrence (KL) grade 4 vs. KL grade 2 OR 21.8; $p < 0.0001$). Risk factors for THR include obesity and heavy manual work.[25]

WHO SHOULD BE REFERRED FOR TOTAL JOINT REPLACEMENT?

TJR is an effective but expensive intervention.[26] Although results from TJR in OA are generally excellent, outcomes do vary, with a measurable perioperative death and morbidity rate, and a small number of patients suffering continuing pain and disability despite replacement.

Currently, there are no evidence-based indications for TJR in OA. Consensus-based criteria for who should get TJR have been produced in the US,[27] Canada[28] and New Zealand.[29] The US National Institutes of Health (NIH) consensus was derived from the opinions of a 13-member panel, 27 experts and a conference audience of 425. Their conclusions were that candidates for elective THR should have moderate to severe persistent pain, disability, or both, not substantially relieved by an extended course of non-surgical (medical) management. The New Zealand criteria also reflect pain and disability, with a maximum severity score of 100. Cut-off scores of 43 and 55 have been suggested;

Table 8.5 Pain and disability associated with New Zealand scores of 55

Characteristic	Maximum	Cut-off at score 55	
		Description	Points
Degree of pain	20	Moderate to severe	14
Occurrence of pain	20	Regular at night	20
Walking ability	10	Able to walk for 11–30 min	4
Functional limitations (e.g. putting on shoes, managing stairs)	10	Moderate limitations	4
Pain on examination	10	Mild	2
Other problems such as reduced range of movement, deformity, limp	10	Moderate	5
Other joints involved	10	None	0
Ability to work, give care to dependants, live independently	10	Threatened but not immediately	6
Total	100		55

55 is preferred and the degree of pain and disability associated with this score is indicated in Table 8.5.

Using such criteria, it is possible to estimate the population need for TJR. It is important to note, however, that this crude measure must be modified to allow for the fact that not all subjects will be fit for surgery, others may not have had an adequate trial of non-surgical treatment and others may simply be unwilling to undergo surgery. Using the New Zealand criteria, Frankel *et al.* estimated a population prevalence of hip disease severe enough to require surgery of 15.2 (95% CI: 12.7, 17.8) per 1000 aged 35–85 years.[30] This equates to an overall requirement in England of 46 600 operations per year; the actual provision is about 43 500. The number of hip replacements currently being performed in England and Wales is therefore approximately correct.

For TKR, the situation is different. Juni *et al.* estimated an annual requirement of TKRs in England, based on New Zealand scores alone, of 55 800 (95% CI: 40 700, 70 900), contrasting sharply with an annual provision of 29 300 actually observed.[31] However, when patient willingness to undergo surgery was considered, this estimate decreased considerably. This study also reported that patients with knee disease were less likely than those with equally severe hip disease to have been referred to a specialist, to have consulted an orthopaedic surgeon or to be on a waiting list for joint replacement. This suggests a perception that TKR is less successful than THR, and that severity should be higher before TJR is considered.

Individuals undergoing TKR vary widely in pre-operative severity of pain and disability.[32,33] Whilst all groups show improvement in terms of function at 3 months, greatest benefit is observed in those with lower baseline disability. There is, therefore, a potential trade-off between operating (on more people) at lower levels of disability, as those patients achieve greatest benefit, and limiting surgery to those fewer patients with more severe disease, accepting that some of their disability may never recover, even with TJR. Geographic variations suggest that this determinant is already operating; patients in Australia having TKR have lower disability than those in the US, with those in the UK being most disabled at the time of surgery.

If patients are asked who should get TJR, they report that priority should be based on length and degree of suffering ('area under the curve for suffering'), pain severity, immobility, paid employment, payment of National Insurance contributions and caring for dependants.[34,35] In contrast, patients think what actually happens depends on age and weight, excessive complaining and access to private practice. It seems logical to take these views into account when planning priority for TJR. Some elderly patients regard pain and disability as an inevitable association of ageing, and may regard themselves as 'undeserving' of TJR. Other barriers to TJR include reluctance by general practitioners to refer, and reluctance by surgeons to operate.

Finally, it is appropriate to consider an economic argument. Health services are limited, and choices have to be made, but these should be made with equity and fairness. One approach, for example, would be to estimate which patient groups have most to gain from TJR. A recent study (K. Payne, L. Davis; personal communication) indicated that patients felt that eight factors should influence access to service provision: pain and mobility, age, cost to the NHS, co-morbidity, ability to return to work, weight and lifestyle, caring responsibility and willingness to take responsibility for one's own health. The perception that it is not unreasonable to direct health-care services to those able or willing to modify their own health has clear political and public health implications.

PREVENTION OF OSTEOARTHRITIS

The risk factors for large-joint OA are becoming well understood. Whilst some (race, gender, age, genetic predisposition) are impossible to change, others are potentially modifiable, raising the possibility of primary prevention.[36] Individuals at high risk of incident knee OA include: those with obesity; a family history; evidence of 'generalised OA', as manifested by the presence of nodal OA in the hands; a history of injury; and a high-risk occupation.

Obesity is a major risk factor for the incidence and progression of knee OA and, to a lesser extent, hand and hip OA. Weight reduction has been shown to be disease modifying. Whilst weight reduction is part of all guidelines for the management of lower-limb OA, strategies to reduce the community prevalence of obesity might also reduce the incidence of OA; conversely, the rapid rise in obesity in most Western countries has major implications for the community burden of OA in the future. Tackling obesity in the general population requires major public health initiatives, and is likely to be achievable only by a combination of reducing intake (changing what we eat – particularly what our children eat) and increasing energy expenditure by promoting aerobic exercise. Again, exercise is beneficial in established OA, but may also have a role in primary prevention; quadriceps weakness is a risk factor for the development of OA.[37]

Repetitive adverse loading of the knee (during occupation or extreme competitive sports) is another potentially avoidable risk factor.[38] Occupations involving heavy physical work, especially prolonged kneeling and squatting, have approximately twice the risk of knee OA. This risk interacts with that of obesity, so that individuals with a body mass index (BMI) ≥ 30 who also have occupational risk factors have an OR for developing knee OA of about 14.[39] Not only is the risk of OA increased but, once an individual has OA, the combination of intense physical activity at work and a high BMI significantly increases the risk of undergoing TKR.[25] In this high-risk group, therefore, it would be possible aggressively to support weight reduction, or indeed avoid obese individuals performing such jobs. Alterations in work practice, by avoiding prolonged work in high-risk postures or using supporting knee pads, may theoretically reduce OA.

Injury – for example meniscal damage at the knee – is a powerful, potentially preventable risk factor for later OA. The role of alignment, joint laxity and nutritional status is less clear.

CONCLUSIONS

There is evidence for a range of surgical and non-surgical interventions in peripheral-joint OA, and health-care professionals involved in managing patients can legitimately be positive about the chances of improvement.

Although new therapies are actively sought, most patients probably do not currently receive the best of what is already available. The main focus remains lifestyle modification. Guidelines have been helpful in providing a critical review of available evidence but do not reflect practice in the real world, where interventions are made in combination, and are limited by local constraints. Important questions to be answered include:

(1)   What drives a medical consultation? Why do some individuals elect to seek medical care?

(2)   What is the effect of pain on the disease process? What would be the effect of early aggressive pain control on allowing better function, activity and muscle strength?

(3)   Conversely, is pain in any sense good, or protective? Would reduction of pain have any long-term negative consequences?

(4)   How can we better identify those individuals at high risk of progression?

(5)   What is the relationship between pain severity and its importance to patients?

(6)   How much risk would patients with OA be prepared to take to achieve a reduction in symptoms?

Many advances have been made in the treatment of OA over the past 20 years. Further developments will depend on:

(1)   Individualizing treatment;

(2)   Better use of available therapies;

(3)   Tailoring therapy to individual needs;

(4)   Better education of GPs and undergraduates;

(5)   A higher profile for OA with 'product champions' informing and helping set the health-care agenda

Management of OA is a truly multidisciplinary task, and the wishes and expectations of the patient should be paramount. Remember: 'Doctors pour drugs of which they know little to cure diseases of which they know less into human beings of whom they know nothing' (Voltaire).

Acknowledgement: The contributions of Professor Paul Dieppe and the Medical Research Council Health Services Research Collaboration to this chapter are gratefully acknowledged.

References

1. van Saase JL, van Romunde K, Cats A, et al. Epidemiology of osteoarthritis: Zoetermeer survey. Comparison of radiological osteoarthritis in a Dutch population with that in 10 other populations. Ann Rheum Dis 1989; 48: 271–80

2. van Baar ME, Dekker J, Lemmens J, et al. Pain and disability in patients with osteoarthritis of hip or knee: the relationship with articular, kinesiological and psychological characteristics. J Rheumatol 1998; 25: 125–33

3. Altman R, Asch E, Bloch D, et al. Development of criteria for the classification and reporting of osteoarthritis. Classification of osteoarthritis of the knee. Diagnostic and Therapeutic Criteria Committee of the American Rheumatism Association. Arthritis Rheum 1986; 29: 1039–49

4. Holdcroft A. Recent developments: management of pain. Br Med J 2003; 326: 635–9

5. Davis M, Ettinger W, Neuhaus J, et al. Correlates of knee pain among US adults with and without radiographic knee osteoarthritis. J Rheumatol 1992; 19: 1943–9

6. Hawley DJ, Wolfe F. Depression is not more common in RA: a 10 year longitudinal study of 6153 patients with rheumatic disease. J Rheumatol 1993; 20: 2025–31

7. Dexter P, Brandt K. Distribution and predictors of depressive symptoms in OA. J Rheumatol 1994; 21: 279–86

8. Yelin E, Lubeck D, Holman H, Epstein W. The impact of rheumatoid arthritis and osteoarthritis: the activities of patients with rheumatoid arthritis and osteoarthritis compared to controls. J Rheumatol 1987; 14: 710–17

9. de Bock GH, Kaptein AA, Touw-Otten F, Mulder JD. Health-related quality of life in patients with osteoarthritis in a family practice setting. Arthritis Care Res 1995; 8: 88–93

10. Leventhal EA. Reaction of families to illness: theroetical models and perspectives. In Turk DC, Kerns RD, eds. Health, Illness and Families: A Lifespan Perspective. New York: Wiley, 1985: 108–45

11. Sanders C, Donovan J, Dieppe P. The significance and consequences of having painful and disabled joints in older age: co-existing accounts of normal and disrupted biographies. Sociol Health Illn 2002; 24: 227–53

12. Croft P, Lewis M, Wynn Jones C, et al. Health status in patients awaiting hip replacement for osteoarthritis. Rheumatology 2002; 41: 1001–7

13. Scott DL. Guidelines for the diagnosis, investigation and management of OA of the hip and knee. J R Coll Physians 1993; 27: 391–6

14. Hochberg MC, Altman RD, Brandt KD, et al. Guidelines for the medical management of OA. Part I. Osteoarthritis of the hip. American College of Rheumatology. Arthritis Rheum 1995; 38: 1535–40 (Updated: Arthritis Rheum 2000; 43: 1905–15)

15. Pendleton A, Arden N, Dougados M, et al. EULAR recommendations for the management of knee osteoarthritis: report of a task force of the Standing Committee for International Clinical Studies Including Therapeutic Trials (ESCISIT). Ann Rheum Dis 2000; 59: 936–44

16. Jordan KM, Arden NK, Doherty M, et al. EULAR Recommendations 2003: an evidence based approach to the management of knee osteoarthritis: Report of a Task Force of the Standing Committee for International Clinical Studies Including Therapeutic Trials (ESCISIT). Ann Rheum Dis 2003; 62: 1145–55

17. Chard JA, Tallon D, Dieppe PA. Epidemiology of research into interventions for the treatment of osteoarthritis of the knee joint. Ann Rheum Dis 2000; 59: 414–18

18. Chard JA, Dickson J, Tallon D, Dieppe PA. A comparison of the views of rheumatologists, general practitioners and patients on the treatment of osteoarthritis. Rheumatology 2002; 41: 1208–10

19. Felson DT, Zhang Y, Hannan M, et al. Risk factors for incident radiographic knee osteoarthritis in the elderly: the Framingham Study. Arthritis Rheum 1997; 40: 728–33

20. Dieppe P, Lohmander S, Falkner A, Chard J. Total hip and knee joint replacement for osteoarthritis. Clinical Evidence. London: BMJ Books, 1999

21. Buckwalter JA, Lohmander S. Operative treatment of osteoarthrosis: current practice and future development. J Bone Joint Surg 1994; 76: 1405–18

22. Merx H, Dreinhofer K, Schrader P, et al. International variation in hip replacement rates. Ann Rheum Dis 2003; 62: 222–6

23. Dixon T, Shaw M, Ebrahim S, Dieppe P. Trends in hip and knee joint replacement: socioeconomic inequalities and projections of need. Ann Rheum Dis 2004; 63: 825–30

24. Tubach F, Baron G, Dougados M, et al. Predictive factors of total knee replacement due to primary osteoarthritis (abstract). EULAR 2003; OP0031

25. Flugsrud G, Nordsletten L, Espehaug B, et al. Risk factors for total hip replacement due to primary osteoarthritis. Arthritis Rheum 2002; 46: 675–82

26. Callahan CM, Drake BG, Heck DA, et al. Patient outcomes following tricompartmental total knee replacement: a meta-analysis. J Am Med Assoc 1994; 271: 1349–57

27. NIH consensus conference: Total hip replacement. NIH Consensus Development Panel on Total Hip Replacement. J Am Med Assoc 1995; 273: 1950–6

28. Naylor CD, Williams JI. Primary hip and knee replacement surgery: Ontario criteria for case selection and surgical priority. Qual Health Care 1996; 5: 20–30

29. Hadorn DC, Holmes AC. Education and debate: the New Zealand priority criteria project, part I: overview. Br Med J 1997; 314: 131–4

30. Frankel S, Eachus J, Pearson N, et al. Population requirement for primary hip-replacement surgery: a cross-sectional study. Lancet 1999; 353: 1304–9

31. Juni P, Dieppe P, Donovan J, et al. Population requirement for primary knee replacement surgery: a cross-sectional study. Rheumatology (Oxford) 2003; 42: 516–21

32. Dieppe P, Basler HD, Chard J, et al. Knee replacement surgery for osteoarthritis: effectiveness, practice variations, indications and possible determinants of utilization. Rheumatology 1999; 38: 73–83

33. Lingard EA, Katz JN, Wright RJ, et al. Kinemax Outcomes Group. Validity and responsiveness of the Knee Society Clinical Rating System in comparison with the SF-36 and WOMAC. J Bone Joint Surg (Am) 2001; 83: 1856–64

34. Woolhead GM, Donovan JL, Chard JA, Dieppe PA. Who should have priority for a knee joint replacement? Rheumatology 2002; 41: 390–4

35. Wright JG, Rudicel S, Feinstein AR. Ask patients what they want. Evaluation of individual complaints before total hip replacement. J Bone Joint Surg 1994; 76: 229–34

36. Felson DT, Zhang Y. An update on the epidemiology of knee and hip osteoarthritis with a view to prevention. Arthritis Rheum 1998; 41: 1343–55

37. Slemenda C, Brandt KD, Heilman DK, et al. Quadriceps weakness and osteoarthritis of the knee. Ann Intern Med 1997; 127: 97–104

38. Felson DT, Hannan M, Naimark A, et al. Occupational physical demands, knee bending and knee osteoarthritis: results from the Framingham Study. J Rheumatol 1991; 18: 1587–92

39. Coggon D, Croft P, Kellingray S, et al. Occupational physical activities and osteoarthritis of the knee. Arthritis Rheum 2000; 43: 1443–9

Index